SHE'S NOT AN OLD LADY WITH DEMENTIA SHE'S MY MOTHER

OUR JOURNEY OF LOVE, LAUGHTER, MUSIC, AND ICE CREAM

Carol Luttjohann, MA, MSW

All rights reserved. No part of this book may be reproduced, stored, or transmitted in any form, mechanical, electronic, or otherwise, except by express written permission of the author. Printed in the United States of America.

The information and events are from my point of view and are factual. However, when multiple people experience the same event, they each can have a different perspective.

There are two chapters credited to the writing being done by my dog, Clancy. Clancy is a Border Collie mix and quite intelligent. However, liberties were taken to give the chapter his voice, but the stories and information are factual.

Copyright © 2013 Carol Luttjohann
ISBN-13: 978-1492277873

DEDICATION

For Mom and Dad

Dad never gave up on Mom. He showed true commitment, love, and sacrifice to keep Mom home where they were able to stay true to their vow: In sickness and in health 'til death do us part. Mom was incredibly inspiring to many until her final day of life on earth. She remained exactly who she had been all her life. And that is why the title of this book is *She's Not An Old Lady With Dementia She's My Mother*.

Deanna Miles

Deanna was one of Mom's hospice nurses and a good friend. She brought sunshine to Mom's life.

ACKNOWLEDGEMENTS

This book is written to honor the memory of my beautiful, wonderful mother. It was my goal through the journey of caregiving to have fun and keep her happy. I succeeded - most of the time.

We met many people on the journey that have left an impression on me. Some were good. Some were not so good. And some were downright awful.

I changed a few names and identifying specifics in telling the stories, but the message remains. It was important to tell some of the worst experiences in order to understand our journey.

I also know there were many we met along the way that considered me a major pain. I saw my primary role as being sure Mom got the highest quality of care possible. I considered getting a t-shirt with "I will be the daughter from hell if you do not take good care of my mother" on it. I never had the t-shirt made, but I lived it.

Thanks to the friends and neighbors who helped with Mom. Fleda and Jim Puck, Teri Rogers, the "boys" next door (Luke, Braden, Garrett, Steven, and Alex) Janet Mitchell, Ruth Newman, and Deanna Miles stayed with Mom so I could run errands and so much more. Sandra Heyman listened to my stories.

Thanks to the many friends who read emails and Facebook posts during my journey and provided encouragement along the way. They laughed and cried with me along the way.

Special thanks to Stephanie Gutierrez and Deanna Miles who read my work in process and provided feedback and honest reactions to help make this a more meaningful and rewarding experience.

TABLE OF CONTENTS

Chapter	Title	Page
1	Introduction	1
2	Ice Cream	5
3	Friends in the Mirror	13
4	Speech Therapy	23
5	Never Too Old	35
6	Mom & Clancy: Part 1	45
7	Mom & Clancy: Part 2	59
8	Mom & Clancy: Part 3	69
9	Cute, Challenging, and Spoiled	79
10	Singing and Dancing	87
11	Seven Months	97
12	You Are So Beautiful	107
14	Imaginary Friends	121
15	Trips Near and Far and Everything In Between	129
16	Lucky Daughter Special Moments	141
17	Afterwords	161
	About the Author	169

HOW TO READ THIS BOOK...KINDA

Chapters are topical and not in a chronological order. Therefore, there is some repetition. There are sporadically boxes with a tidbit about things I learned that I hope will be helpful.

There are also sections between chapters what I call "Mom-isms". A "Mom-ism" is a fun or special moment with Mom – things she said and did.

The last chapter is filled with "Mom-isms" from our last sixteen months together on earth.

She stayed the same wonderful, feisty lady all her life. She did not change personality. She lost mobility only because of arthritis. She kept smiling right up until the very last moments of life. And she never stopped asking for ice cream.

I miss her.

> Mom told one of her imaginary friends we would help them. I said, "I have enough to do taking care of you."
>
> She reached up, patted me on the cheek, and said, "You are so cute."
>
> January 2012

> Mom <to friend>: Where's Carol?
> Me: Here I am, Mom.
> Mom: Be quiet. I am looking for Carol. Oh, you are Carol.
> September 2010

> I warmed up one of the soft blankets for Mom. I put it over her and asked if she liked it. Big Mom smile. The smile is worth it all. I had another blanket warming in the dryer. Little Momma was happy and healthy.
>
> August 2012

INTRODUCTION

I am the fourth of five siblings born to Leo and Claudia Luttjohann. From oldest to youngest: Sherry, Kathy, Leo, Jr., Carol (me), and John.

We lost John to suicide on January 16, 2003.

There are also nine grandchildren and nine great-grandchildren.

A harsh reality is caring for elderly parents can be difficult, and conflicts arise. I chose to help keep my parents at home where they wanted to remain. Unfortunately, there was substantial conflict between Dad and my siblings. I do not know all the details, and I am not sure it matters. The end result was my siblings making the decision to not have contact with Mom and Dad beginning in the summer of

2008. That meant the grandchildren and great-grandchildren also stopped contact.

I was in graduate school at Washington University in St Louis from early 2007 to the middle of 2008 when everything transpired. I returned to my hometown of Topeka, Kansas after finishing my Master of Social Work and dove into caregiving.

My original plan was to get Mom and Dad set up, comfortable, and able to remain at home. I was then going to work on getting full time employment around the end of that summer.

However, that fall Dad was diagnosed with a blood clot, then lymphoma was found in early 2009. He died August 24, 2009.
When Dad died, despite having had no contact with Mom for over a year, my siblings wanted to move her to a nursing home. She said she did not want to go. I supported Mom's decision and was able to keep her at home until she died.

Sherry and Kathy saw Mom a few times over the next three years and three months. Kathy usually had her grandchildren with her. The rest of the family chose not to be a part of Mom's life.

She died November 29, 2012.

Details and analyzing the situation are not important. My siblings, and therefore, the grandchildren, and great-grandchildren made the decision to not be a part of Mom's and Dad's lives. It was their choice and definitely their loss.

This book is a gift for the younger family members. They missed being a part of the life of their grandparents. These are the stories that shape them.

The joy Mom brought to my life and so many others is the focus of this book.

> Mom was telling me a story. She said, "She was pretty young – maybe 40 to 70."
> June 2010

> Mom got cleaned up and went into the TV room where Dad was watching sports.
> Dad smiled and said, "You smell nice. I like clean old ladies."
> Mom replied, "And I like dirty old men."
> Summer 2009

> The podiatrist says Mom's feet are in good shape. Circulation good, etc. He said her feet are in better shape than patients half her age with diabetes. It's obvious she has managed her diabetes, took care of herself, and that I am doing a good job caring for her now.
> June 2010

Carol Luttjohann

ICE CREAM

It's all about ice cream. Mom's favorite food was ice cream. Any ice cream. Anywhere. Any time.

Mom announced she was going to fix supper.

"Great," I said. "What are we having?"

"Ice cream."

I took the hint and told her I would get her some ice cream.

"You can have some, too. You take a little, but give me a lot."

Mom even mastered eating ice cream in her sleep. She asked for ice cream. I went and got some for her. When I returned, she was lying down.

"Do you want your ice cream?" She opened her mouth. After she had finished about half the bowl without ever opening her eyes, I asked, "Is that enough?"

"No." She opened her mouth.

She finished off an entire bowl of ice cream without ever opening her eyes.

One day in early January 2010 we had had a very busy day. We had been on the go a lot. After supper, Mom laid down and fell asleep. It was about 7:00 pm. She was sleeping soundly until 11:15 pm. She woke up, sat up and said, "I have been sound asleep, but I woke up when I remembered I have not had any ice cream."

There was no such thing as a day without ice cream for Mom.

It was not unusual for Mom to have a second supper. She needed enough carbohydrates to sleep through the night without low blood sugar. And sometimes she was just plain hungry.

One night after her second supper, which she devoured, she asked for ice cream. I got some for her. She was getting very drowsy.

I asked, "Are you tired?"

"That's why I am closing my eyes."

But, she opened her mouth. It was another masterful evening of eating ice cream while she was close to sleep.

We had a lot of fun with her love for ice cream.

One day when she was sleeping a lot she woke up and asked for ice cream. There was nothing unusual about that.

While I was feeding her the ice cream she said, "You are a good girl."

"Do you like ice cream?"

She giggled and responded, "You are funny."

After she finished the ice cream, I put a warm blanket on her – straight from the dryer. I loved doing that for her.

She said, "Oooooooooooohhhhh that is nice. Good night." And fell back asleep.

I kept a rotation of warm blankets on her during cold weather. A full night's sleep was a luxury. I napped when I could. But keeping her warm and happy was the goal.

She ate well most of her life, but she did have moments of stubbornness.

I was feeding her a grilled cheese sandwich, beets, and peaches for supper. All of a sudden she stopped eating. She closed her mouth.

"Do you want some more?"

She kept her mouth closed and did not respond.

"Are you still hungry?"

No response – just a tight lipped Mom.

"Are you waiting for ice cream?"

The wonderful beautiful Mom smile filled her face.

She had been very quiet for the past couple of days, so it was even more wonderful and something to celebrate. I fed her a bowl of ice cream.

"This is the last bite."

She ate it and opened her mouth. She finished a second bowl, and then opened her mouth again waiting for more. She ate three bowls of ice cream before falling back asleep.

Although three bowls was not the norm, it was not uncommon.

One day in late 2009, she told me she needed to eat three bowls of ice cream so she could gain three pounds. I was never sure why three pounds, but I do know why she wanted ice cream!

There was a family that lived near my old house – I had moved out of it to move in with Mom and Dad to care for them. The family has six kids. The youngest four came to see Mom once in a while. They came and filled the house with energy and laughter and ate ice cream with Mom.

The only boy was 8 years old at the time. He would sit and hold Mom's hand while waiting for his turn to play Wii. All of them loved Mom.

The last summer Mom was living, I got her out one evening and went to the youngest girl's soft ball game. She was 7 at the time. We stayed for about an hour and a half and watched one inning of the game.

The kids all came over to Mom to tell her good-bye. The 7-year-old girl could never remember Mom's name. She said, "Good-bye. I love you, Carol's mom."

After Mom died, I took all the ice cream that was left in the freezer to the kids. I am sure she smiled when she saw a bunch of energetic children enjoying ice cream. She always did.

> Mom loved having the children visit and going to see them. And, like Mom, they loved ice cream.

> When I was feeding Mom tonight, she said, "You are such a good girl. I love you."
> I wasn't even feeding her ice cream.
> March 2012

> Me: Are you glad you are my mom?
> Mom: I think so.
> August 2011

> I fixed Mom a wonderful dinner with cole slaw, potato salad, mixed vegetables, and fruit. Mom ate a couple of bites and asked, "Do we have any ice cream?"
> January 2012

I took Mom to a non-emergency clinic. It was one we went to often enough they knew her.

We needed to get a referral to a neurologist.

The Physician's Assistant left to go get the appointment set up. When she returned, Mom said, "What took you so long?"

The PA responded, "I'm sorry it took me a minute to do that."

Mom immediately said, "A minute!? We need to teach you to tell time."

March 2010

I took Mom to run errands.

Me: Do you want to stop and eat lunch or go home and eat?

Mom: Okay.

Me: Eat out or go home. Pick one.

Mom: One

October 2010

FRIENDS IN THE MIRRORS

"Leo, there's someone in the house."

Dad got up out of his comfortably padded lawn chair. He was sitting on the screened-in back porch, which was one of his favorite hobbies, to go check the house. The birds, rabbits, and squirrels would have to wait for their daily feeding of seeds, crackers and bread crumbs.

He had spent three years in the Army Air Corps in World War II – one and a half years overseas. When he returned home, he spent a little over 20 years managing Luttjohann Crushed Stone, Inc., which his dad owned. After that he worked for the State of Kansas in areas of accounting until he retired.

In 2004 he had a stroke and depended on a cane for walking. He still drove some, was dedicated to watching Jeopardy, Who Wants to Be a Millionaire, Wheel of Fortune, and any kind of sports. He also habitually kept up with the national and world news via CNN.

For local news he read the newspaper daily and watched local broadcasts. He did the newspaper crossword puzzles every day.

He and Mom were married in 1943, and now 65 years later he was a caregiver. Mom had been diagnosed with dementia. She also had diabetes and arthritis.

At 87, he had earned the right to sit and relax. But he also was completely dedicated to Mom. So he grabbed his cane and headed to the door with Mom close behind.

They went through the kitchen, turned right into the television room, a left turn took him out into the hall. They made their way through the hallway, opening and closing the hall closet door and a quick check of the bathroom.

They arrived at the end of the hall and

checked the front bedroom, turned back into the all and made a right turn to go into the living room. A quick scan of the living room, noting the front door was locked, and then turned left into the dining room and back to the kitchen. They had made the full circle and checked everywhere.

Dad knew when he got up they would find no one, but he also knew the importance the simple task of walking through the house had for Mom.

The few minutes investigating put Mom at ease.

Paranoia is not uncommon with dementia, but in hindsight I wonder if Mom was seeing people in the mirrors. She always seemed to see "those people" in the hall and front bedroom – both had mirrors.

She no longer recognized pictures of herself, and it could have been as simple as seeing herself in the mirror and not knowing it was her.

Another common characteristic of dementia is not recognizing oneself.

Mom not recognizing herself in the mirror actually became common as time went on. She stopped seeing people in the mirrors as strangers or people to fear. And instead began to make friends with all of them. Her conversations with her friends in mirrors provided insight into how she was doing, but also a lot of laughter.

When she was in physical therapy, there was mirror used for patients to provide visual feedback on use of limbs. Not applicable for Mom's therapy, but when she saw the mirror, she stopped and talked to her friend. She smiled and laughed.

Every time she went to physical therapy, she stopped to visit with her friend.

"Hi. It's good to see you again."

Short pause as she waited for a response. friend.

Tim, the Physical Therapist, worked well with Mom. He found it difficult to communicate, but he was able to help Mom with balance. And he helped me to understand ways to help Mom with exercises and lots of walking. He would patiently wait long enough for Mom to have a brief conversation then encourage her to move on.

"Claudia, let's go work with the balls," he would suggest.

Mom understood and told her friend, "I need to go. Come see me sometime," she would say motioning a come-with-me kind of gesture. One of the times Mom stopped to chat with her friend, Tim asked, "Would you like to go for a walk?"

Mom replied, "No, thanks. You go ahead. I will watch."

Tim told me how cute and sweet my mom was. He also told me I was a saint for caring for her.

Mom had many friends in mirrors. At home, her friend in the hall mirror she called Mary. Mary was her confidant. When Mom was upset or frustrated she often talked to Mary and then she felt better. I encouraged her to talk to Mary when she was upset. It always seemed to help. Mary was a good listener. And I was able to listen in and find out more about Mom and help her.

Then there was Tom. Tom was in the mirror in Mom's bedroom. Tom was nice, but more of a casual conversationalist. Although one day when we were going to run errands, Mom said Tom wanted to go. So the mirror had a place on the backseat of the car safely strapped in the seatbelt. Tom could be a good friend to have around, but he had a side that was a bit ornery.

One day I was in the living room, and I heard Mom in her room. She was very angry with Tom. When I went to investigate, she said, "Look at what he did," pointing to a bowl of ice cream sitting on the floor. "I gave him that ice cream, and he threw it on the floor."

I did not dare laugh knowing how angry she was at Tom for his mischievous deed. Instead I picked up the bowl of ice cream, handed it to Mom, and said, "Why don't you go ahead and eat it? Tom doesn't need any if he is just going to drop it on the floor."

Mom and I retreated to the living room leaving Tom alone to think about his mischief.

Anywhere there was a mirror, Mom found a friend.

During a lengthy wait in a doctor's examining room, Mom was becoming restless and fidgety. It happened sometimes. I simply placed a chair near the door and sat in it. There was no reason to do anything other than let her have the freedom to walk around and fidget. But I also guarded against her leaving the room.

Then, she looked towards the back left corner of the room. Her eyes lit up. She went to the mirror, leaned towards her new friend in the mirror and said, "Come on, let's you and I get out of here." She was heading towards the door as the doctor came in.

Although Mom no longer recognized herself in the mirror, mirrors were important to keep her company. They were wonderful friends – as long as they did not throw ice cream on the floor.

Watching the progression of dementia was not easy, but it was not without opportunities to laugh and enjoy. The choices were allow Mom to be who she was, build on the strengths, and enjoy every moment or see changes as failures and give up on her.

Giving up was never an option.

Getting past expectations of what she "should" be – what she was in the past – and instead loving and appreciating the moment is important in caring for someone with dementia.

It didn't matter if Mom put her shirt on over

her nightgown, declared she liked those clothes and wore them to the grocery store. It didn't matter if she ate oatmeal with her hands when she had difficulty using utensils.

Stuff did not matter.

Mom and her friends in the mirrors did.

> People with dementia appearing to be paranoid and seeing people that are not there might be simply seeing people in mirrors. Take down the mirrors or cover them and see what happens. Or you might try introducing them to the person in the mirror…they might make a new friend that likes car rides. But most of all do not give up on them. Life is short for all of us, and your life will be greatly enriched if you take time to allow people to be who they are.

> Christmas 2011 we had a cookie decorating party. I baked a lot of cookies. Some broke, so Mom and I were eating them.
>
> Mom: Those are good.
>
> Me: There's the buzzer. I have to get more cookies out of the oven.
>
> Mom: Break some. They are good.
>
> December 2011

> I took Mom to visit Kathleen and Karen tonight. She was able to stay for 1 ½ hours. A year ago we might have been able to stay about ten minutes.
>
> June 2010

SPEECH THERAPY

I took Mom to a neuropsychologist in January of 2009. He did a lot of testing and evaluating. He diagnosed aphasia, which is the partial or total loss of the ability to articulate ideas or comprehend spoken or written language. He did some specific testing for dementia. His testing eliminated what I already believed. Mom did not have Alzheimer's. Her difficulties stemmed from multiple mini-strokes caused by lengthy episodes of high blood sugar. There were other medical professionals who said they could not tell Mom was diabetic from her feet, which they usually can. Also, the Podiatrist said Mom had the best looking feet of all of his patients. He said he had patients half her age that had been diagnosed with diabetes within the last year which did not have such healthy feet. It would have been impossible for her to have such healthy feet if her diabetes had not been controlled for the most of the more than 40 years she had lived with diabetes.

However, after John died in January 2003, Mom had a lot of difficulties (no surprise). Her diabetes was out of control. The two were connected. If the first line of defense had been to manage the diabetes, it is a possibility she would have had fewer cognitive problems. Instead her diabetes was sporadically out of control, and she had multiple TIAs (mini strokes) over a period of probably four or five years.

It was not until December 2009, after a ton of research and after Dad's death, I got Mom to speech therapy. Speech therapists work with cognitive skills, including aphasia.

Although Mom was not able to analyze and understand making the decision to go to Speech Therapy, she could understand what I explained to her. I talked to her about how it could help, what would happen, and involved her in making the decision. She wanted to try.

I looked into various options and found a therapist near where we lived.

We went to the first appointment. It was an initial consultation and evaluation. Ellen, the Speech Therapist, was forty-something and had a lot of experience. She began her normal evaluation process. She needed to get a baseline for Medicare. There had to be progress for Medicare to keep paying for therapy, so the starting assessment of abilities was important.

Among the tasks was for Mom to read a card and answer the question on the card. Simple enough. Mom was doing quite well. Then she read the card, "How many ears does a man have?"

Ellen asked, "Can you answer that question?"

Mom responded, "How many ears does a man have?"

"Yes."

"It depends on his mood."

Ellen counted it as a correct response.

The next set of tasks was Ellen reading directions for Mom to follow.

Again, overall, Mom was doing quite well.

Ellen said, "Point to your chair."

Mom responded, "My chair is at home."

Ellen tried, "Nod your head."

Mom did not respond.

I asked, "Can you nod your head?"

"If you want it done, do it your own self."

After the initial visit, I waited in the lobby area and let them work. I stayed close by in case I was needed. Sometimes towards the end of the hour session, when Mom was getting tired, I would go in and help.

I started bringing cookies, candies, and juice for Mom. When she was getting bored, Ellen would give her a short break – eat a cookie, take a drink. That's all it took for Mom to get back to work.

Over a fairly short time, just a couple of months, Mom made substantial progress. She was reading, answering questions, following two stage commands – things like stand up and touch your nose – and more. Her problem solving skills were improving. Ellen kept moving her to more and more complex tasks.

Identifying objects is a skill that is easily lost with dementia – the searching for the name of what that thing is.

Ellen held up a screwdriver and asked, "Does this have a name?"

"I'm sure it does."

"I guess I did not ask what the name of this thing is."

Ellen then put three objects on the table and said, "Hand me the pencil."

"Say please."

"Please hand me the pencil."

Mom handed Ellen the pencil.

They sang songs. Mom could sing along. They sang Happy Birthday to me a lot. Singing is good for rhythm and speech patterns.

Reasoning and analytical skills began to improve.

Ellen asked, "Who might say, 'Three strikes, and you're out.'?"

"Carol."

Close enough.

"Who might say, 'You owe $10.27.'?"

"Someone I would tell to go to hell."

Mom mastered that level.

One day Mom was not very responsive. Ellen asked, "What are you thinking about?"

Mom replied, "Well I am having a debate with myself, and it is not going very well."

Having mastered, the who-might-say level, she moved from following directions to read the directions on the card and follow the directions.

There were more and more complex tasks.

I was sitting outside the door listening.

Mom was tired of the game. She had had another appointment before Speech Therapy. She was getting tired and hungry. Not a good combination. I went to help get her through a few more cards.

We did two or three more.

Then Mom picked up a card, looked at it, and said, "It says, 'Go home with Carol now.'"

She looked at me and said, "Let's go," and headed for the door.

She truly mastered the level. She understood what the "game" was and was able to manipulate things to get what she wanted. Ellen was very impressed. After just a couple of months, Mom had done a lot.

She had gone from an initial evaluation of 30, at six weeks she hit 70, and by the time we stopped, she was getting 100 frequently.

Soon things leveled off. She made slower progress, but continued. About nine months into Speech Therapy, Mom told Ellen, "You keep asking me the same things."

It was true. She was. But Mom had reached a plateau and was having difficulty going much further. It was time to stop. There was no reason to continue just to continue. I had learned a lot about what to do and how to help her. I continued writing things down for her so she could read and understand.

We made labels for things in the house so she could read them.

We wrote short stories, cut paper shapes, followed simple directions to make arts and crafts.

She was not going to regain all that she had lost, but I could help her keep trying and maintain as much as possible.

Anything that helped her with problem solving was also part of the routine – which shirt do you want to wear – pink flowers or blue stripes? Limiting choices to what she could manage.

Asking her to make decisions – problem solving.

We had a garden and were going to give some of the vegetables away. It was a very small crop of four small green peppers and two tomatoes. I asked, "Do you want to give these to Judy or Kathleen?

It was a difficult question. Judy, a nurse, who lived next door neighbor helped Mom and understood what was going on with her. Kathleen is Mom's sister-in-law. They had been friends for over 60 years.

Mom thought for a moment, then replied, "Half to each."

Each of them got a tomato and a couple of green peppers.

Another day I asked, "What do you want to do today?" I listed four options. She pondered the question a moment. Then she said, "Write them down, and then I can pick one."

Simple ideas. Simple solutions. These kinds

of things do not sound like much. But to me and Mom they were mountainous. It was allowing her to make decisions, to think about choices that made a difference even into the final weeks of her life.

A little over two years after she had stopped speech therapy, there was evidence at how much it helped her retain and maintain skills.

She continued to make decisions and problem solve. Mom died on a Thursday. The day before, on Wednesday, I said, "How about oatmeal for breakfast?"

Mom smiled and replied, "How about ice cream?"

She had ice cream.

I often said aging parents are the gods' revenge for our teenage years.

Elderly want their independence. They want to make choices about where they live and how. Mom had always said she wanted to remain in her own home. She did. But it also was important to ask her questions about she wanted to eat, what she wanted to do, and involve her in decisions. I talked to her about everything. It could makes things more difficult or more time consuming to involve her in choices. But it was worth it.

She kept her dignity.

> There were times when Mom would not sleep or was restless. It was her way of letting me know she needed something. On one occasion when she was not sleeping, I first tried giving her a drink. That did not work.
>
> She was dry and clean. I tried oatmeal – a usual favorite. Then French toast. Finally I tried a fresh baked chocolate chip cookie.
>
> She happily ate it and said, "This is much better."
>
> October 2012

> I got Mom up and into her wheelchair. I took her into the bathroom for a "shower."
>
> I put several layers of blankets (hospital white) and towels on the floor to absorb the water – usually enough. However, today Mom said how good the warm water felt and was rubbing herself to work up a lather with the soap herself. HUGE MESS. But worth it. She felt clean and was trying to do it herself. It was worth the mess and extra laundry.
>
> September 2012

NEVER TOO OLD

"I don't need to know how old old is because I am never going to be old," Mom declared.

Claudia Jean McIntosh made her debut into this world on April 1, 1926. She was born in Osage City, Kansas. Her original birth certificate lists her mother as Josephine Frances Berry (aka Grandma Francie). No father is listed. In 1935 a new birth certificate was issued listing Robert Hazlett McIntosh as her father. There is a note on that birth certificate saying it was issued after "Robert adopted Claudia."

One time my brother, John, asked Grandma Francie what she would have named Mom if she had been a boy. She replied, "Eddie Lee."

John said, "I'm glad she was a girl. I would hate to have a mom named Eddie Lee."

One day Mom told me she was going to live to be 123 years old. I told her if she lived that long she was going to have to start taking care of me. She agreed.

She was always quick with comebacks when I did refer to her as old.

We were regulars at Golden Corral. Mom loved the buffet.

I would order for us, "Two. One old lady and one not as old."

Mom always quickly added, "I am the not as old."

Then we would choose a table, and I would go fill plates and bring them to her. Maybe that is why she loved it. She got to sit and watch, and I would wait on her.

One of the tasks I had was to order an omelet for her. Tammy made the omelets. I ordered a vegetarian specialty of mushrooms, onions, and jalapenos. Then Tammy would bring the omelet to the table and kiss Mom on the cheek. Mom beamed. She loved feeling so special.

Mom would devour the omelet.

After we finished eating, we would stop to say good-bye to Tammy. She would leave her place behind the omelet table and give Mom a hug.

Our last trip to Golden Corral was just about three months before she died. We selected our table. Everyone knew her and talked to her while I grabbed plates of food. Only now I had to feed her.

She still devoured every bite of her omelet.

Mom loved outings, and a favorite place was to visit Aunt Kathleen and her daughter, Karen. Karen was Kathleen's daughter – the only girl of the five children Kathleen had. Karen lived with and helped care for Kathleen.

One evening as we were leaving, Mom was still very mobile. She was taking her time as we went to the car. I said, "Come on, Old Lady."

Mom immediately replied, "I am old, but I

can still fight."

It was rare she acknowledged being old, but when she did it was a feisty admission.

On one of the occasions Mom had blood work done, the nursed poked Mom's left arm, and the needle popped back out. She tried Mom's right arm. And again the needle popped back out.

As the nurse was about to try again, this time she as going to put it in her hand, Mom said, "You better get it right this time. I am an old lady, and I do not tolerate nonsense."

In 2009 we celebrated Mom's 83rd birthday.

I fixed lunch for her and several of her friends.

We had frittatas, asparagus with almonds, fruit, and of course, ice cream.

It was several months later I slipped and made a comment about Mom being old.

Mom: I am not old.

Me: You are 83. That isn't old?

Mom: No. My dad is older than I am.

Me: That's true. You are my mom, and you are older than I am.

Mom: But you are getting older.

Me: So are you.

Mom: But you show it more.

She never lost the quick wit and wonderful comebacks.

In 2010, we took apple pie and ice cream to Kathleen's house and celebrated with Kathleen and Karen.

April 1, 2011 was a major date for Mom. It was her 85th birthday. I wanted to do something that would be special for her. We celebrated all weekend. Her actual birthday was on Friday that year.

I took Mom on a short road trip to Kansas City. It's a little over an hour drive to Oak Park Mall there. We went to Build A Bear. We used her wheelchair. She was very able to walk, but I took the wheelchair when there was going to be a lot of walking. She would push the chair. If she got tired got tired, she could sit, and I could push the chair.

I was not sure where in the mall the Build A Bear store was, and it turned out I parked at the wrong end of the huge mall. We had a good jaunt to make it there. Mom was in the chair by the time we got there.

We looked around and asked about building bears for her birthday. When the clerks learned it was Mom's birthday, they gave her a big "It's My Birthday" sticker to wear. Mom's big beautiful smile said it all.

The first step in the process was to choose a bear or one of the other animals to stuff. I took Mom to see the huge wall of choices. She wanted a bear. When I asked if she wanted to make a boy or girl bear, she paused, thought, and wrestled with the idea. Then she proclaimed she wanted one of each.

She chose a white bear to be a girl, and a

brown bear was the boy. We took them to the stuffing machine. The clerk asked her to choose hearts for her bears. There were several choices. Mom studied each carefully, picked them up, looked at them, and finally decided on a plain red one for the boy and a red with white polka dots for her girl bear.

Next she could choose to add sounds. The devices were put in their paws. When squeezed, the boy says, "I love you," and the girl plays, "Braham's Lullaby."

The bears were filled with stuffing and stitched closed.

Next came choosing clothes.

I helped narrow choices to two outfits for each.

Mom's final decision was a pair of grey shorts for the boy with a blue plaid shirt. He also got heavy brown shoes – they remind me of ones Mom's dad used to wear.

The girl has a pretty pink, purple, and white

plaid striped dress with yellow sparkly lines. A pink ribbon belt with a daisy and pink bow decorate it. She has pink sandals with flowers on her feet. One of the clerks brought Mom pink bows and helped put them on the girl bear's ears. Mom loved them.

Last in the process was to create birth certificates. After a lot of debate and discussion, she decided to name them Robert and Frances after her parents.

Robert and Frances accompanied us to breakfast at Golden Corral that Saturday morning. Kathy and her husband met us there as did some friends. The crew there, who loved Mom dearly, sang Happy Birthday to her.

Sunday Robert and Frances kept watch as we had a small open house. Mom talked to her bears sometimes. She loved to hear Robert say, "I love you" and Frances play Braham's Lullaby. They sat on her bed and were with her the rest of her life.

In 2012 we had a celebration for her 86th birthday. It had been just a few weeks earlier the physical therapist had helped me start getting Mom out of bed more often.

I made a butterfly cake, and we set up the party in the front yard. Sherry and Kathy came.

So did Ruth (Mom's long- time friend) and her daughter, Patsy. Patsy and Sherry were the same age, and of course, because our moms were friends, we had spent a lot of time together growing up.

Several friends and neighbors came by. Kathy's grandkids were there. They played and enjoyed being outside. The two great granddaughters held Mom's piece of cake with a candle while we sang Happy Birthday. It was a wonderful, but very exhausting day for Mom.

Her bears, Frances and Robert, from last year's birthday were still her favorite birthday present. She held them, talked to them, and slept with them, and they kept watch over her.

She continued to protest being called old. Just a short month before she died, I told her, "You are my sweet old mom."

She immediately replied, "I am not old." However she was never too old to "play with" her special teddy bears.

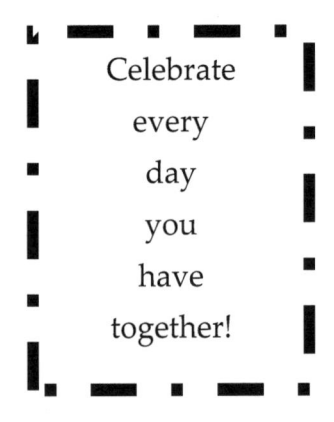

> Celebrate every day you have together!

Carol Luttjohann

MOM & CLANCY: PART 1

About a month before Dad died in 2009, I started spending nights at my parents' house. Until then I had been there 12 to 14 hours a day. I was at home at night. In the early days of caring for them, it was not unusual for Dad to call me to come back because Mom was having difficulties. Typically when she was having anxiety or other problems it was related to recalling traumatic memories. Talking through her memories resolved a lot of problems. In 2008, when I first began the caregiving role, Mom's diabetes was out of control, and she was having frequent urinary tract infections. It was the diabetes and urinary tract infections causing problems. I began, first, getting Mom off the slew of medications she was on. It was difficult to tell what was happening with her because of the massive side effects of medicines. It did not take long to get her on just one medication for diabetes. I managed everything with diet, exercise, activity, and time with her.

When we first started walking, we would go out the back door, down the alley about 2-3 houses, then return home. Over a few weeks we worked our way to being able to walk a mile every morning and every evening. This was critical to manage the diabetes.

It took a while to figure out Mom was becoming dehydrated, and that was what was leading to the urinary tract infections.

I added unflavored Pedialyte to her drinks. A mix of about 1/3 Pedialyte and 2/3 juice produced results.

She went from a urinary tract infection almost monthly to two or three in a year.

Mom also had traumatic memories we dealt with. Having a lot of patience and help from Dad, I was able to talk her through them and turn the traumas to good memories. I was able to give a different perspective on what had happened that helped her see things differently.

One reoccurring incident she talked about is asking what happened to the little boy. Mom had had three major incidents in her life that I knew about, involving losing a little boy.

The first was during my parents' first year of marriage, Mom had had a baby boy that died. I don't know any more details than that, but Mom did talk about the baby that was taken away, and they never talked about him again. I am not sure if it was the baby or not.

A second little boy was one Mom's mother, Grandma Francie, had told us about. Mom was an only child, but at one time Grandma Francie and Grandpa Robert were going to adopt a little boy. Grandma Francie said when the depression hit, they were afraid they would not be able to take care of him, so they did not adopt him.

It was not until Mom had memories of this

that I understood more. With some prodding and asking questions and adding what little I did know, I got this story from Mom:

There was a little boy that lived with them. Her dad took him and put him in the car because the other people could take better care of him. The kicker was when she said he reached for her hand, but she did not take his. That is when he was taken away.

Mom was maybe three or four at the time. And the little boy was a toddler under two.

The memory had stayed with her. She was haunted by not taking his hand. She thought if she had taken his hand, she could have saved Him, and he would have stayed with her.

It was also not until we worked through that story that I found out the little boy had actually lived with them for some time. I am not sure how long they had him, but it stayed in her mind.

The third little boy story was when my

brother, John, died. He was 46 and not a little boy. However, he was the youngest of the five of us siblings. He was Mom's baby boy. Although there was nothing specific in talking about losing John, it was clear that she thought she should have been able to save him.

We lost John to suicide on January 16, 2003. Tragic no matter what. But that was three major "little boy" losses. We really only spent a lot of time on the little boy that was taken and given To another family - the almost adopted little boy.

After that "session," it was over a year before she mentioned a little boy again…..it was when Dad died she asked, "Where's my little boy?" It was only once. It was the day after Dad died. Just long enough for her to realize he was gone, but the whole idea had not truly sunk in.

There were other traumatic memories we worked through, but soon resolved them. One involved Mom talking about abuse she experienced during her short stay at a nursing home in 2007. It was more than six months after the fact, but she was very afraid of talking and of "those guys."

Because it had been so long and she had dementia, it is unlikely anything could have been done. But Dad and I assured her she would never be in a nursing home again. We promised to care for her at home where she would be safe.

The traumatic memories became much less prevalent as her diabetes got under control, and she was off of all but the diabetes medication. I never believed I could actually "cure" Mom. But I was sure I could help her regain and maintain some of what she had lost. And by 2009 when Dad was diagnosed with lymphoma, Mom was doing much better. She still had bouts of problems, but they were fewer, farther between, and much more manageable – simply going for a walk worked wonders. And by 2010, after some work in Speech Therapy, she was making decisions, problems solving, and doing even better. She was not without problems, but substantially different than she had been in 2008.

I was 24/7 with both of them beginning July 19, 2009. Dad tended to sleep days and want to be awake at night. Mom slept nights and was awake during the day. I am not sure when I was awake or asleep, but I got through the last weeks of Dad's life caring for both of them.

Dad had not tolerated my dog, Clancy, being around, so Clancy had had to spend a lot of time alone. He visited and spent time with us, but it was not until after Dad died Clancy moved to Mom's house with us. Three of us. Mom, Clancy, and me.

Clancy is my dog. I got him when he was just six weeks old. Mom went with me to get the puppy. I found him through a free ad in the newspaper. It was a free ad for puppies that were half Border Collie.

He is what many call tan and white, but his color reminds me more of the red color in a collie – like I remember Lassie from TV fame. He has a lot of white on paws and chest. His white marking on his face looks like half of an hour glass. He also has one brown eye and one blue eye – and the brown has a tiny spot of blue on it.

Border Collies with wide white markings are on their faces are more likely to have the bi-color eyes.

His human birth mom said Clancy's dad looks like a collie.

The neighbors call him Prince Charming – that translates to Clancy has a lot of brothers and sisters. The best guess is Clancy is Border Collie and either Husky or Aussie mix. Either way he is gorgeous and smart.

When I walked in the house to see the puppies, I immediately went to Clancy. I fell in love with him the moment I saw him. I held him for a while, and then put him down so I could see the other puppies – all boys. I got down on the floor. About that time their mom came into the room. All the other puppies ran to her to nurse. Clancy stayed right with me. He was the one.

When we got in the truck to take him home, Mom cradled him and sang to him on the drive home. They also connected immediately.

When I moved Clancy full time to live with us, Mom already had developed a strong protective nature of the dog.

Clancy's middle name is Jasper, and I frequently call him CJ. Mom's name is Claudia Jean. The same initials. I think it was an omen of some kind - a good one.

The first night he was there I was sitting in the pink rocking chair by Mom's bed watching television and eating. Mom was in the recliner. Clancy jumped on the bed and was eagerly eyeing my plate of food. I put my arm up to hold him back so I could eat.

"Don't you hit my dog," Mom said.

"I didn't hit him. I just put my arm up to hold him back while I eat."

"You hit him. Apologize to that dog."

I apologized to the dog.

A few days later as I was walking by Clancy on the bed, he jumped off the bed, landing on my bare foot. I reacted, "Ow, that hurt."

Once again the wrath of Mom came.

"Don't talk to my dog like that. Apologize to him."

I complied.

It became obvious that a certain dog had Grandma wrapped around his little paw. I was the outsider. Their bond was strong.

Mom loved having the dog go for walks with us. Clancy seemed to understand Mom's needs and would walk slow enough so Grandma, as she referred to herself, could take her time.

When I fixed ice cream for Mom, Clancy also had a bowl of ice cream. He had plain vanilla.

He would pick up his bowl and carry it to wherever Grandma was and sit with her to eat ice cream. Mom, very protective of her ice cream, would still share with him.

Clancy soon developed a taste for whatever ice cream Grandma was eating. If she was too slow, he would put his paws on the snack tray And help himself while she was finishing her bowl of ice cream. Not the most sanitary conditions, but when I tried to intervene, I was admonished to apologize to the dog for daring to suggest he not eat out of Grandma's ice cream bowl.

Mom started giving him bites of ice cream. She would drop a spoonful on the floor for him. Clancy caught on quickly and would catch ice cream mid-air.

Their sharing soon included all meals. Clancy initially got leftovers. But soon mastered the art of stealing bits and pieces of things off Mom's plate. Intervention was hopeless. He could take a single potato chip off her plate without touching anything else on the plate. Mom did not care, and I simply gave her seconds, thirds, whatever it took for her to get full and avoid apologizing to the dog.

One day I fixed her a snack of peanut butter and crackers. I put it on the snack tray and went to the kitchen to get her a drink. When I returned, there were only two crackers left on her plate where there had been 10.

I looked at Clancy. He knew there was nothing I could or would do. Mom ruled. She was okay with sharing, and if I took action, I would only have to apologize for my daring to say anything negative to the dog.

There he sat in the middle of the living room floor with a smirk on his face and peanut butter on his breath.

Clancy had been with us for almost two years enjoying ruling the house with Grandma at his side. But then I started finding occasional puddles.

Disappointed, thinking Clancy was having problems with what had been successful housebreaking, I would find a puddle, and put him outside.

Soon I found the puddles were actually another sign of Mom's progression. She had entered what I affectionately dubbed the pick a place to pee phase.

She was still making it to the bathroom frequently, but other times she was not. It was a step between fully able to tend to her own needs and incontinence. It was going to require being more attentive to what she was doing and keeping Mom on a schedule for bathroom breaks.

It wasn't easy to find Mom was responsible for the puddles and not Clancy. It meant adaptions, changes, and another level of caring for Mom. Before the tough work with Mom could begin, I first had to apologize to the dog.

Pets are very important to keep close by. Clancy is a gentle soul and was wonderful to have with Mom. They had a very special relationship.

MOM & CLANCY: PART 2

Mom and I took care of Grandma for a long time. We loved taking care of Grandma. She had dementia, diabetes, arthritis, and all kinds of other things we had to help her with.

I know Mom already told you about me, but this is my version. My name is Clancy Jasper. Mom named me after the dog she had before me. His name was Jasper. My dog mom is a Border Collie, and no one is sure about my dog dad. He looks like a collie, but Mom thinks I might be part Husky or Aussie. It doesn't really matter. I am adorable no matter what. I am orange-tan color with white markings. I have one blue eye and one brown eye. My brown eye has a little bit of blue on it. Mom says the white marking on my face looks like half of an hour glass. When she tells me stuff like that, I just bat my eyes.

Mom and Grandma saw an ad in a newspaper for free puppies. That is how they found me. Mom walked in the house and picked me up. I loved her immediately.

She started to look at my brothers, but they all ran to see our dog mom when she came in the room. I stayed with Mom and Grandma. I picked Mom and Grandma. I let her think she picked me. Dogs know who they are supposed to live with and take care of. We have special jobs, and I knew the moment I saw them Mom and Grandma were my people to take care of.

They needed me.

While Mom drove the truck home, Grandma held me and sang to me. She was tone deaf, but I did not care. She loved to snuggle, and I liked that. I was not quite six weeks old.

I lived at Mom's house with her for nine months, but then we had to move to Grandma's house. Grandpa died, and Grandma needed help all the time. I loved it. Grandma was a lot of fun.

Mom already told you about how Grandma used to make Mom apologize to me. We started things off right that first night I stayed with Mom at Grandma's house. Mom was learning Grandma and I were in charge. Grandma and I had already spent a lot of time together, and she did sing to me on the way home from my dog mom. I had Grandma wrapped around my little paw.

Mom and Grandma and I liked to go for walks sometimes. I had to walk slowly when Grandma walked slow and could walk fast if Grandma did. Grandma needed special care, and it was my job to help her. When Grandma could not walk by herself, Mom put her in the wheelchair and held Grandma's hand so she could sit in the chair and walk. When Grandma's arthritis got bad, and she could not bend her legs to sit in the chair, Mom made a special thing for the wheelchair with electrical conduit. Grandma could sit in the chair and keep her legs out on the thing Mom made. We kept going for walks. Grandma loved being outside.

One day, when Grandma could still walk a lot, Mom was mowing the lawn.

Grandma was on the back porch and I was on my long leash out back. Mom went to mow the front yard. When she did Grandma got up and started to walk towards the alley. She was walking down the ramp on the back of the house, and as soon as she got where I could not reach her, I started barking really loud. Mom came running. Grandma was just taking something to the trash can out back, but Mom was glad I watched Grandma so carefully. I wanted to be sure someone was there to help me keep an eye on Grandma.

Once Grandma fell and bumped her head. Mom was worried. Grandma seemed to be okay, but Mom called the paramedics. Mom wanted to be sure Grandma was okay since she bumped her head. The paramedics said Grandma was supposed to stay sitting down. I went and put my head on her lap until the paramedics got there so she would stay safe.

My job was to protect her. It was really nice. Grandma kept petting me. She loved to snuggle with me. The paramedics took her to the hospital to have her checked out. She had an infection. But she was okay.

When Mom fixed ice cream for Grandma – Grandma loved ice cream – she gave me a bowl of plain vanilla. I would pick up my bowl and carry it to wherever Grandma was and sit with her and eat ice cream. Sometimes we sat in Grandma's chair. Sometimes we got on the bed and ate ice cream together. Grandma always shared her ice cream with me- well, almost always. If she was too slow, I would help myself to her bowl of ice cream. Mom told you about that.

Sometimes Grandma would get mad at me. She did not like it if I got too excited and barked a lot. She would tell me, "Be quiet, ass hound." Mom and I thought it was funny, but I stopped barking because I knew Grandma meant it when she said that.

When Grandma could not walk and stayed in her bed a lot, one day there were a lot of flies in the house, and they kept swarming around Grandma. So I got up on her bed and laid down beside her. Whenever a fly came near her I snapped at it and caught it. It took a while, but I stopped all the flies from coming to sit on Grandma. I was so tired after all that work, I stayed on the bed, and Grandma and I took a nap together. Mom took pictures.

We also liked to sit on the porch. Mom would take bread, crackers, and seeds out into the yard for the rabbits and squirrels and birds. Grandma and Grandpa used to feed them, too.

Grandma loved to watch the animals. Mom always told me not to chase them and let them eat. So I did.

One day I saw a little rabbit in the yard. I went and lay down on the sidewalk and watched him. Finally he hopped away. Then I went and smelled where he had been. Mom told me I was a good dog. She said, "Clancy, you are a gentle soul.   You take good care of Grandma and you take good care of the rabbits."

I told her, "Of course I take care of the rabbits. Rabbits are dogs, too."

Grandma died in November 2012. I miss her a lot. I miss going for walks, eating ice cream, and snuggling with her. I am lucky to have had a Grandma to love so much and who loved me. And I love taking care of Mom now.

She gets sad sometimes and misses Grandma.

So we snuggle and talk about her. I do a lot of listening.

And I give Mom special kisses right on her nose – that's her favorite.

And once in a while she even apologizes to me, but she never calls me ass hound.

> Another note on pets... I let Mom and Clancy interact however they wanted as long as Mom was safe. She had times when she let him eat with her and times she did not. It was her choice.

> Mom absolutely refused to go into the bathroom for a shower with a bath aid.
>
> She had a bed bath – the aid did the best she could sitting by Mom on the couch.
>
> Aid: You sure are being stubborn today.
>
> Mom: What's your point?
>
> December 2010

> Me: Mom, you are hilarious.
>
> Mom: So are you. That's why we have so much fun.
>
> August 2010

> Mom said she was cold. I gave her a blanket, which she promptly put over her head, covering her tent-like.
>
> From under the blanket I heard, "It's hot in here."
>
> March 2011

> Bath Aid: How are you today?
> Mom: I'm just fine. How are you?
> <later nurse arrives>
> Nurse: How are you today?
> Mom: I haven't decided yet.
> November 2012

> When we went to the grocery store, I told Mom to stay with me because I did not want to explain to anyone I lost my mother.
>
> She replied, "I saw your mother last night, and I did not see anyone who looked like they were lost."
>
> April 2011

Carol Luttjohann

MOM & CLANCY: PART 3

My name is Clancy Jasper. I am the adorable Border Collie mix dog that helped my mom take care of my grandma. We had a lot of fun, but it was not all easy. Mom was pretty challenging at times. She still is.

Mom liked to fix things and make things for Grandma. She was pretty clever.

Dogs know who they are supposed to be with and take care of. I knew immediately Mom and Grandma were my people. And I loved taking care of Grandma. Although sometimes I had to be a bit creative about how I approached her. But I could always count on Grandma to share food with me and keep Mom in line.

One day she finished eating so I jumped on the bed bedside her. She rearranged the food on her plate so it would be easier for me to reach. When I finished she said, "I dropped a little on the floor over there. You might want to jump down and eat it, too." Of course I did!

She always made sure I got all leftovers.

One time Grandma finished eating and Mom was taking her plate and asked Grandma if she wanted more. Grandma said, "No." Then she looked at me and said, "Do you want more? She can get you some if you want more." I got SECONDS!

I loved Grandma so much.

One time Grandma would not eat supper until Mom fixed a plate for me, also. We had lentils and potatoes. They were pretty good Mom gave Grandma some baked beans, but she would not let me have any.

Another time Mom made quiche. She left me and Grandma alone. When Mom came back, I had the quiche on the floor eating. She asked Grandma if she wanted more. She did, and she told Mom to bring me some more. I loved that wonderful lady.

Sometimes she would eat most of her food and only share a little with me. But she almost always told Mom to get me more.

And Mom always did because if she did not do what Grandma said, Grandma would make Mom apologize to me.

One day I was trying to eat some of her food, and she took her plate and held it up over her head and yelled at me to stop.

Mom came to check on us, and I had to go in the other room so Grandma could eat. Mom did not have to apologize for that. And when she was done eating, she would let me clean off the plate. She made sure I got plenty to eat.

Grandma was not always good about sharing ice cream. Sometimes she did, but sometimes she did not – like when she was eating ice cream, when she stopped, I helped myself to her bowl. Grandma got really mad.

She yelled, "Stop! That is mine, you ass hound."

I was laughing so hard I almost did not make it to my favorite tree.

She called me ass hound when I took the stick after she ate a fruitsicle. That was okay. It was funny.

Grandma loved to go outside on the porch. So Mom would get Grandma in her wheelchair and take her out on the porch.

Then the nurse, Deanna, said Grandma needed to keep her legs up so she should not sit in the wheelchair for very long. Grandma was having problems with edema. That means her legs would swell up, and that was not very comfortable for Grandma.

But Grandma liked going outside so Mom decided to build a bed for Grandma on the back screened in porch.

Mom took some 2x4s and built some tiny wall looking kinds of things. She measured everything so it would be easy to move Grandma from the wheelchair to her bed. She left room on one side so she could put the power lift under it. Then she had Daniel make the door between the kitchen and the dining room wider so Mom could get Grandma in the lift and roll her all the way to the back porch and put her in the outdoor bed.

Then my clever Mom used electrical conduit and fixed Grandma's bed so Grandma could sit straight up, or kind of recline or lay down flat. And she put a ceiling fan outside on the porch.

We spent a lot of time on the porch. Grandma loved being outside. Mom would sit by her and talk to her about the birds and squirrels and rabbits.

But the fun part was when Mom built some shelves. Grandma and I were in the house when Mom decided to move them, but the cat, Delilah, was on the porch. When Mom moved the shelves, she bumped the ceiling fan and the shelves started to fall. That cat was bouncing around and running. She looked like a furry ping pong ball.

I was laughing and had to run fast to get to my favorite tree.

I helped entertain Grandma, and Mom entertained me with her power tool antics.

One time I put her on power tool restriction and hid all of her tools. I put them under the bench on the front porch. It was a day Aunt Deanna was coming to visit. I sent her an email and made her promise not to tell Mom where the tools were. I gave her an extra bottle of Coke – her favorite drink – for helping me.

Mom put me in charge of protecting Grandma. Mom helped, but I was in charge.

There were a couple of times Grandma had some surgeries for cataracts and also she had to have a colonoscopy to be sure she was okay. Mom said when she took Grandma to have the cataracts remove, the nurses told Mom to take good care of her "very sweet mom." That's my grandma! Very sweet and very loved. Mom and I did take good care of her.

Grandma always slept a lot after she had procedures, and I would sleep on the bed with her. And when I had to get neutered, Grandma had an urinary tract infection, too, so we slept on the bed together and helped each other. Mom says we were very cute. We took care of each other when we were sick and when we were healthy.

Grandma liked me to give her kisses when she went to bed, and I was always glad to do it. I could usually get a taste of ice cream when I kissed her.

I liked to bite at Mom's feet just for fun.

Mom said, "Why are you biting my feet?"

Grandma said, "He likes feet."

Another trip to the tree for me.

My very favorite was when Mom filled the bath tub and put some stuff in it to make bubbles. She left the bathroom to get towels and clean clothes. When she came back, I was in the bath tub. I had bubbles on my chin.

Mom and I were with Grandma when she was dying – the last minutes of Grandma's life. We knew we were not going to have much more time with her. Mom held Grandma, and I stayed by her so she could see me. Grandma smiled at us. She was not afraid. Dogs know. I am sure Grandpa was there to help Grandma. He always did take care of her and loved her. That is why Grandma was not afraid.

Just a couple of minutes after Grandma died, our friend, Ruth, came over. Ruth was trying to get there before Grandma died, but did not make it. Ruth and Grandma had been friends since they were in Junior High. Ruth cried. I sat by her so she could pet me. It made her feel better. I liked it, too.

Mom let me go outside to wait for Aunt Deanna. When I saw her, I barked and dug the ground and jumped a lot. I was telling her how glad I was she was there to help me with Mom.

Aunt Deanna talked to Mom and told her what a wonderful person Mom is. She said Grandma was lucky to have Mom take care of her. Mom said she was the lucky one.

I miss Grandma, but I am glad I got to help take care of her even if it did mean I had to make a lot of trips to my favorite tree.

> Mom: If you don't know the answer, just keep talking until someone tells you, then agree.

> Mom's eyes are closed. I could not tell if she was sleeping or not.
> Me: Are you awake?
> Mom: <eyes closed) No.
> November 2012

> Mom: Is your mother coming over today?
>
> Me: You are my mother.
>
> Mom: Then I am glad I came by.

> I took Mom for a drive and stopped and got some ice cream for her. As we were on the way home she said, "I'm cold." She paused a couple of seconds then added, "But that is probably because I am eating ice cream.
>
> Note: About two years and four months earlier (March 2008), she could barely walk. Her blood sugars were soaring, and she was not very verbal. Diet, exercise, eliminating unneeded medications, and socialization made a huge difference!
>
> July 2010

CUTE, CHALLENGING, AND SPOILED

Mom: What should I do today?

Me: You can sit there and look cute, but that might be too hard for you.

Mom: Nah, I am really good at that.

How true! Mom was a master at being cute. She could also be challenging. She had a quick wit and great comebacks. She was feisty and stood up for herself.

I went to her side of the car to help her get out. She asked, "Am I supposed to get out?"

"Yes. Unless you have a strong emotional attachment to your seat belt."

"That was funny. Did you read that in a book?"

In four and one-half years of caring for Mom, I cannot even count the number of people we encountered that fell in love with her. She was adorable and very sweet.

In November 2009 she had her first cataract surgery. She woke up the morning of the surgery. Her appointment was at 12:30 p.m. She was not going to go completely under anesthesia, so she could eat whatever she wanted.

She woke up at 4:30 a.m. and ate a vegie omelet, hash browns, and toast. She went back to sleep, woke up at 8:30 and had pancakes and fruit topping.

Around 10:30 I gave her some ice cream and asked, "You have already had two breakfasts and now you are eating ice cream. Why are you so spoiled?"

She responded, "Because I said so, and I am in charge."

I took her for her surgery. She was out of sight, and I was nervous. The nurse came to ask me questions about her health.

She asked, "What has she had to eat today?"

I laughed and told her the long list of food Mom had had.

When they brought her out after the surgery, the nurses told me to take very good care of my very sweet mother.

No problem.

I always asked Mom what she wanted, what she wanted to do, and worked at involving her in all decisions. We were out running errands.

"We are going to stop at the store. Do you want anything?"

No answer.

"Do you want anything at the store?"

No answer.

" Mom, are you ignoring me?"

"Yes."

" You're driving me crazy."

"That's not my fault. You were already like

that."

There was a few minutes of silence.

"I'm thinking."

Mom immediately said, "You're thinking! That's unusual. We need to celebrate."

She could be very challenging when trying to communicate – not listening was an art she mastered well.

Another outing she asked, "What are we doing?"

"Running a couple of errands, then your Speech Therapy, then a picnic in the park."

She was obviously not paying attention.

"Are you listening?"

"Yes."

"What did I say?"

"Are you listening?"

And one of my absolute favorites.

We were running errands. "We need gas."

Mom immediately said, "Huh?"

I practically yelled, "We need gas."

"You don't have to yell. I am not deaf."

"It seems like everything I say you say huh or what."

"Go to hell. See I don't just say huh or what."

Clancy helped with spoiling Mom. He took good care of her.

In the fall of 2011 we had an abundance of flies in the house. Mom did not tolerate my swatting flies on her bed. It scared her.

Clancy solved the problem.

The 45 pound dog parked himself at the head of the bed – just above Mom's head and snapped at flies that came by her. He stayed until they were all gone.

Late in 2010 a chaplain that visited Mom came by. They sat and talked. Mom loved singing with him. When he sang, "How Great Thou Art," Mom sang every word with him.

Then he said, "Let's pray together."

Before he could say anything, Mom began, "God, take care of us…"

Faith was very important to her. She told me in early 2011, "I know things can be hard for you, so I am praying for you."

Mom always stayed in charge. Although she did tell me I could be in charge to do whatever she told me to do. She also said I could live with her as long as I did not do anything to make her mad.

Spoiling her and Mom being cute went together. I helped her get on a shoe. I started to help with the second one. I stopped and said, "You can do this yourself."

She stuck her foot out in front of me and said, "Why?"

Even as time progressed, she never lost her quick wit and sense of humor.

I was feeding her a chocolate chip cookie. She was happily eating and said, "This sure is good."

"You sure are cute," I replied.

She laughed and said, "You got that right."

Because of Mom the house was filled with laughter – both her laughing and smiling and laughing with her.

The blessings were many during those years.

> I offered Mom a Hershey's Hug. She opened her mouth, and I put it in. As I did, she closed her mouth and bit my finger. I yelled, "Ow."
>
> Mom said, "That was fun. Let's do it again."
>
> October 2012

> Deanna came to stay with Mom and Clancy while I ran errands.
>
> Deanna told Mom, "You raised a wonderful daughter. Carol is a good person. She loves you and takes good care of you."
>
> Mom responded, "I know."
>
> Then she fell asleep.
>
> August 2012

> Affirming Mom's beauty and worth daily gave her strength. She never forgot she was a valuable human being worthy of being treated with dignity and respect.

I made tomato basil soup for lunch. Mom was eating it and seemed to be enjoying it.

Me: Do you like the soup?

Mom: Ice cream would be better..

After she finished her soup, I gave her some ice cream and cookies.

Mom: You are a good woman.

September 2012

Beautiful sunshine day. I moved Mom's bed right by the front door so she could see outside and feel the sunshine. She was semi-tapping her toes to John Denver music.

January 2012

Carol Luttjohann

SINGING AND DANCING

During the four and one-half years I cared for my mother at the end of her life, I lived in her town – Claudia's Place. A special place created for Mom and me to reside as we walked the journey of dementia. Claudia's Place was both real and imaginary. It was real that we were dealing with the progression of the disease. It was imaginary because only Mom and I actually lived there – a place just for us. It was a place where we connected, and it was a place where Mom was safe, secure, and happy. We had visitors from time to time, but only the two of us actually resided at Claudia's Place. A beautiful place filled with love.

An important part of Claudia's Place was music. Mom loved music. She was tone deaf – could not carry a tune no matter what. But she would still sing along with favorite songs. When she was in high school, she wanted to take guitar lessons. Her parents said no because she could not hear the tunes. So Mom got a job and paid for the lessons herself.

During the early days, the bedtime routine was:

Mom would get in bed. I would tell our dog, Clancy, "Tell Grandma goodnight." He would jump on the bed, "kiss" Grandma and retreat to the living room.

Then I would say, "Good night, Mom. I love you." And she would respond, "Good night, Honey. I love you, too."

As I left the room, I would push the button on the CD player and start her bedtime music. Her favorite was the CD *20 Classic Hymns*. As I left the room every night, she was listening to Track 1 on the CD.

When peace, like a river,
Attendeth my way;

Carol Luttjohann

When sorrows like sea billows roll;
Whatever my lot,
Thou hast taught me to say,
It is well, It Is Well With My Soul[1]

In hindsight that song was very appropriate. I had no idea what was going to happen from day to day, but I knew whatever challenges and joys were ahead, Mom and I were in this for the long haul. And it would always be well with our souls. Another favorite was the Statler Brothers, especially their gospel CDs.

Mom and I used to dance to the Statler Brothers music. We danced to a lot of music. One night we were having our own party – just the two of us – at Claudia's Place.

We were listening to *Statler Brothers Gospel* CD, Mom stood up and said, "Let's dance.

So we danced to *His Eye Is On The Sparrow*.

Why should I feel discouraged?
Why should the shadows come?

> *His eye is on the sparrow,*
> *And I know He watches me*[2]

As time progressed and Mom was less able to dance, she would walk in her wheelchair, and we would we dance.

One day I found an old Bing Crosby CD. Dad used to love to sing, and Mom loved listening to Dad sin.

Bing Crosy's *Irish Lullaby* was a favorite.

Mom was in bed listening to the CD. She was quite advanced at this point. Track 8 began and Crosby started to sing:

> *Over in Killarney many years ago,*
> *Me mother sang a song to me*
> *in tones so sweet and low.*[3]

As Mom listened to the music, she raised her very weakened arm up. Reaching her hand towards the ceiling, she grasped an imaginary hand. Her feet began to move as she danced to the music.

> *Too-ra-loo-ra-loo-ral, Too-ra-loo-ra-li,*

Too-ra-loo-ra-loo-ral
That's an Irish lullaby.[3]

The song ended, and she lowered her hand grasping tightly to the imaginary hand and gently kissed it. When *Irish Lullaby* ended, so did Mom's dancing. She quietly continued to listen to the music.

It was one of the most powerful and memorable moments of the entire 4 ½ years.

She was connecting to Dad, and was truly beginning her journey to join him. Now there were three of us residing in Claudia's Place – Dad joined Mom and me. He became very present as we continued our journey of dementia in Claudia's Place.

Over the next year after that, we continued to have music on most of the time. She loved all music. We danced to big band music even when she was in bed. I moved her arms around energetically as we sang and danced to *Chattanooga Choo Choo*. Her beautiful big Mom smile said it all.

Music was very important in Claudia's Place and was part of all of our activities. Singing and dancing – connecting in special ways.

During the last three months of Mom's life, our friend Deanna would stay with Mom when I ran errands. Deanna is also a nurse. She became a resident of Claudia's Place. She was not a full time resident with Mom, Dad, and me, but Claudia's Place was real for Deanna, also, as she walked the journey of dementia with us.

Deanna would put in CDs and sing with them. Mom would sing along with her. One day, after Deanna was gone, I asked Mom if she remembered singing with Deanna.

She replied, "Yes. That was fun."

Music. It was very important to her. She loved to sing. She loved listening to music. She connected to music in many ways and on many levels.

Mom had always liked Peter Paul and Mary

so I had their music on a lot. One day, when Deanna was there, the Peter Paul and Mary music was on. Deanna was singing along with it.

Mom looked up at Deanna and said, "Enough already."

Deanna asked, "Enough of my singing or of Peter Paul and Mary?"

Mom replied, "Peter Paul and you know – what's her name," shaking her finger vigorously at the CD player.

Deanna took the Peter Paul and Mary CD out and put in a John Denver CD. Mom was happy. The song Mom enjoyed the most was *Sunshine.*

That was their song. The song linked them to Claudia's Place.

Early in November 2012, I had an Open House for Mom. Friends and neighbors dropped by to visit her. I did those once in a while to keep her in contact with people. Mom enjoyed having visitors at Claudia's Place. When Deanna and her partner, Chris, came by, we put on the John Denver CD, the *Sunshine* track.

As Deanna sat beside Mom and sang, Mom kept reaching for Deanna's hand and was actively involved in the music. Mom could not always sing with the music any longer, but it was obviously touching something deep within her. *Sunshine* was making her happy. It was lovely to watch her. It made her smile.

The next day I put the CD in again and sang with it. Mom had the same reaction. She was active, reaching, touching her deep within. It was a way she was communicating with us – through her special music.

A little less than two weeks later, Mom took her final breath. Her musical journey in Claudia's Place had gone through many phases. She had gone from being well with her soul to knowing God was watching over her to reaching out to Dad who was helping her prepare for her final journey to letting us know that her journey had been filled with *Sunshine* - filled with happiness and tears, but in the end lovely and filled with highs.

Mom left Claudia's Place on earth and joined Dad in heaven, but Claudia's Place remains very real and very imaginary deep within me…and always will.

---

[1] Spafford, Horatio G., *It Is Well With My Soul,* 1873.(Public domain)

[2] Martin, Civilla, *His Eye Is On The Sparrow,* 1905 .(Public domain)

[3] Shannon, J.R., *Irish Lullaby,* 1944. .(Public domain)

> I gave Mom a foot massage, complete with a warm towel, lotion and followed with chocolate.
>
> Me: I sure do spoil you.
>
> Mom: Keep it up.
>
> September 2011

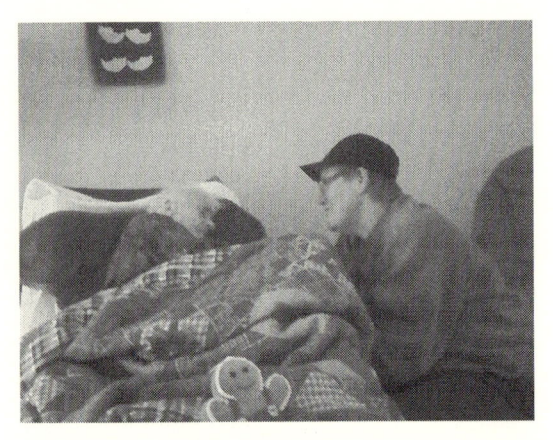

Mom and Deanna listening to and singing *Sunshine*. This was just 12 days before Mom died. A beautiful, touching moment. Mom was telling us it was almost time for her to go. November 2012

SEVEN MONTHS

It's still hanging on the wall in the living room – the dry eraser board I put up to make communicating with hospice workers easier.

The living room was our everything room. Mom and I both had beds in there. I wanted to be close to her, to listen to her, to talk to her. I would sometimes lie on her bed beside her. I would put her bed right beside mine and hold her hand at night. I also set up a kitchenette – a small refrigerator, microwave, and the small chest freezer stocked with plenty of ice cream.

The dry erase board was put up to use for notes, information on how Mom was doing, when nurses, aids, chaplains, social workers, and others would visit. It was all written on the board. I was not incredibly rigid about keeping it up-to-date. All the information that was once here is gone. But one word remains. Claudia.

Written in block letters the C and D are outlined in red and decorated with blue dots, L and I are outlined in blue with black slashing lines, both As are black with green squiggly lines, and the U is green with red smiling faces.

It is still on the wall in the living room, hanging over the antique like dresser where Mom's music players used to be.

There were two – one that looks like an old fashioned record player that plays CDs, records, and cassettes, and another kind of ugly looking oversize radio- almost the size of an old VHS player that plays eight tracks.

The sounds of Statler Brothers, John Denver, Bing Crosby, The Lennon Sisters, Guy Lombardo and many others used to fill the room. But the players are gone now – moved to my computer room / office. That's where the music is now.

But the dry eraser board remains. How long

is long enough to leave it hanging on the wall? It's been seven months since Mom died. Is that long enough? Should I be ready to take it off the wall and put it away somewhere or maybe put it on another wall and use it? I know it is no longer needed for Mom, but how can I use it for something else? And why that board?

Why do I leave it there?

Other things that were unique for Mom are long gone or packed away. Some things were easy to get rid of – leftover adult pull ups. I never used adult diapers for Mom – only pull ups. I had a thing about keeping her dignity. Pullups were normal. Diapers were degrading in my thinking. Mom only had pullups. Some of the over the counter pills and her one prescription for diabetes – Senna, enemas, and Glimepiride are gone. I kept the Advil.

There were pads I kept under her because of her being incontinent – the disposable ones are gone. The cloth ones are washed and packed away. I am not sure why I am keeping them, but they are in a box in the attic.

Clothes. I cut up some of them and made yo-yos to put on a quilt. For quilting a yo-yo is a piece of fabric, cut in a circle, and gathered up…I used them to make butterflies and flowers on a quilt I have on my bed. Some clothes are packed away. Some are in the pile for the garage sale next week.

There were special foods for Mom. I gave the ice cream to the kids that used to come visit her and eat ice cream. They live over by my old house – just a few blocks away. They came over once in a while and ate ice cream and played. Mom loved having kids around. The kids are very sweet and kind. The seven-year-old girl could not remember Mom's name. When she would leave, she would say, "Good-bye. I love you, Carol's mom." And the eight-year-old boy would sit by Mom's bed waiting for his turn on the Wii. He would talk to her and hold her hand.

Those are the kids who got the ice cream. It seemed right. Some other foods I ate. Some I threw away.

The special medical equipment – the bed, the bedside commode, the over the bed table, adaptive things for the bathroom, walkers, wheelchairs– all stored away in the basement. Some things like the lift and the special Broda chair went back to the equipment rental company.

Pretty much everything is packed away, given away, or thrown away. So why not the dry erase board?

Other things that were needed for caring for Mom are gone. The mobile I got for Mom is packed away. I used it daily. I would wind it up and listen it to it play music as Winnie-the-pooh, Tigger, Rabbit, and Eyeore moved around in a circle. Some days Mom would hear the music and watch the mobile move around. Some days she could hear the music, but could not figure out where it was. And some days she acted as if she did not hear it at all. It helped me know how she was doing.

Things that had been taken off the walls to make room for special things for Mom are back. The paintings Audria Young painted.

Audria was seventy-something when she started painting. She won several times in the county fair. Her paintings had been stored away to make room for things for Mom. The painting Audria did of the church in the middle of a field is back. Dad lived near where that church was at when he was young. He recognized it.

The large painting of Topeka – it is a mixture of scenes of downtown Topeka. It was taken down because it was right by where Mom's bed was. I did not want to take a chance of it falling on her. It was behind the piano for a long time. It is a special edition painting.

There used to be two sets of chrome shelves – five shelves on each one – piled with necessities for Mom: nightgowns, towels and washcloths, medicines, medical stuff – like the thermometer, blood pressure cuff, and pulse oximeter were on the shelves.

There were white hospital blankets – most of them were accumulated when Dad was nearing end of life and was always cold. I used to keep the white blankets warm for Dad – a continual supply warming in the dyer, changing the one closest to him every 30 minutes or so to keep him warm in the last couple of weeks of his life. I did the same for Mom – warm blankets for her. She always said, "OOOOO that feels good" when I put a warm blanket on her. There were soft blankets that I used to cover pillows to put under her legs to keep her heels from rubbing on the bed so she would not get sores. I always put the soft side of the blankets so it would be against Mom. I heated those for her also. There were sheets, pillow cases, hair care stuff, and her nail care kit – nail polish, nail polish remover, clippers, files, and cotton balls.

Saturdays were manicure and pedicure day for Mom. I used special soaps I got from Avon to clean her feet. Then I wrapped her feet in towels that I warmed up in the dryer. I used lotion and massaged her legs and feet, clipped her toenails and put on nail polish – she chose the colors sometimes. Then she had hand massages and fingernails clipped and filed. I put polish on her fingernails, too. She also had facials on Saturday – warm towels and special cleansers. She was loved and pampered, and she almost always thanked me for the special care I gave her.

She always smiled.

The shelves and all the contents are no longer in the living room. They are in the garage holding tools and other garage stuff.

How long is long enough to keep a dry erase

board with "CLAUDIA" written on it when everything else is gone?

The DVD player we used is in my computer room. I use it sometimes to play movies while I am on the computer. I used to put it on Mom's over the bed table so she could watch movies.

Her two favorites were *Bridge to Teribithia* and *Young at Heart*. *Young at Heart* is a documentary about a group of older adults from Massachusetts who travel around the world singing rock and roll. Mom loved listening to the music. When a 92-year-old woman started singing, "I feel good …." Mom smiled her big beautiful special Mom smile.

Bridge to Teribithia is a beautiful story of friendship between a young boy and girl. They build a fantasy world, Teribithia, where their imaginations soar and they have many adventures. Mom loved to watch the kids. There is a lot of singing in that movie, also.

The DVDs and the player are gone from the

living room.

But the dry erase board remains. I guess it is somewhat symbolic for some reason. I just do not know why. Maybe it is because it has CLAUDIA written on it. Everything else that was on it is erased.   Maybe it is because I don't want to use it for anything else – it is Mom's.

I don't know how long long enough will be.
But seven months is not long enough.
And that is okay.

> It was just a few weeks after I wrote this chapter, I took down the dry erase board and repainted the living room. It had not been a living room for four years. CLAUDIA is still written on the board. It is still not used for anything else. More time will bring that. Take time to grieve.

Carol Luttjohann

YOU ARE SO BEAUTIFUL

When Mom and her sister-in-law, Aunt Kathleen, worked at Macy's, their day off was Tuesday. Aunt Kathleen worked on the dock. Mom worked in Housewares.

Aunt Kathleen was married to Dad's brother, Henry. So Mom and Kathleen were sisters-in-law and very good friends.

Kathleen used to tell the story about the first time she met Mom. Mom and Dad were already married. They came to visit Kathleen and Henry. Mom brought a dish filled with cookies.

During the summers, when Mom and Kathleen had Tuesdays off, the two of them, my brother, John, and I used to take day trips.

We went to Holton to go swimming. The public pool there had an island in the middle of it.

That was a novelty at the time.

We went to Ottawa to go to antique stores.

We mostly went to small towns for one reason or another.

Mom drove the VW bug. Mom and Kathleen sat in front. John and I were in the back. Mom always drove down the middle of the street. One time Kathleen asked her why. Mom responded if she drove in the middle, she would be ready to turn in either direction.

She was a master at last second turns.

She used this art very skillfully years later when I was caring for her.

We would go to the grocery store. Mom would follow me through the aisles pushing the cart. She always went down the middle of the aisle. That way she was always prepared to run into me no matter which side of the aisle I was on.

Despite the challenges of diabetes, dementia, and so much more, Mom was always Mom. Too often people talk about a loved one with dementia as if they no longer exist. Actually people talk about elderly, who are very much alive, in past tense. The things they used to do and who they used to be.

I could never see Mom as "used to be." Yes, she definitely lost some abilities, and she needed more help than she had earlier in her life, but the heart and soul of Mom remained.

I often said elderly parents are the gods' revenge for our teenage years. Even the "best" of teenagers struggles to find their identity, to have the right to make decisions about their lives, and want independence.

A study commissioned by Clarity and EAR Foundation that was done in 2007 found elderly fear moving into a nursing home and losing their independence more than they fear death.

Dad and Mom had always said they wanted to remain at home. They helped their neighbor, Elmer, stay in his own home. They helped care for him for ten years until Elmer died in his home at the age of 96. They also helped another neighbor, Lydia.

It was Mom's nature to take food, run errands and check on elderly she knew.

Understanding Mom and Dad wanted to stay in their home was only part of why I did.

It was much more.

The Fifth Commandment, the commandment with a promise, says, "Thou shalt honor thy father and mother that your days may be long on the earth." It does not say, Honor your father and mother . . . unless they forget your name or unless you do not like their decisions or any other exceptions.

I did some research on the Fifth Commandment when I spoke at Dad's memorial service.

It's an absolute.

I also found when directed at adult children, the commandment included protecting parents from being driven from their homes.

It is fascinating to me that the greatest fear of elderly today has such deep roots.

Caring for Dad during his last 15 months of life was better for him and Mom because they were together.

Dad and Mom were an awesome couple. I was always amazed they lived together for just shy of 66 years. During that last 15 months they had together, many memories were shared and a lot of laughter.

During the summer of 2008, Mom and I began walking. It was part of keeping the diabetes under control. Exercise is one of the most effective ways to lower blood sugar. But I also baked a lot of apple pies. I did use sugar free apple pie fillings. It was challenging to get Mom walking faster – partly because she had not been active for a while and partly because of arthritis. Dad suggested I put a piece of apple pie on a string and hold it out in front of her to entice her to walk faster.

Dad was amazingly patient and caring with Mom. He said it was part of the secret to their long marriage – being true to their word – he cared for her in sickness and in health. And after such a long marriage, he had learned the value of keeping mama happy. They had a routine.

Dad would say, "If Mama ain't happy…"

Mom would reply, "Nobody's happy."

One day Dad said, "If Dad's not happy, nobody's happy."

Mom quickly corrected him saying, "You better be careful. Mama keeps Dad happy, so if Dad wants to be happy, he better keep Mama happy."

Dad almost swallowed his cigar he was laughing so hard.

Mom had difficulty bathing. One day I helped her get cleaned up – shower, powder, touch of perfume. She went into the TV room where Dad was.

He looked at her and said, "You smell nice. I like clean old ladies."

Mom quickly replied, "And I like dirty old men."

For their 65th anniversary in 2008, Dad took Mom out to dinner. Mom was social and liked to talk to people – whether she knew them or not.

They went to McFarland's and Mom greeted the people in each booth as she passed by them.

It was not easy for him. But Dad saw more value and beauty in Mom and accepted her as she was.

In May 2009 Mom had a reaction to a medication and ended up at the Emergency Room. They kept her overnight for observation. Two major events happened with Dad during Mom's short stay at the hospital.

First since Mom was asleep, I went to check on Dad. We sat on their screened in back porch. With tears in his eyes, he thanked me for helping them and told me if I had not come back to Topeka, he would not have had the past year with Mom.

He said either she would have died, or he would have had to put her in an out of home placement.

It is sad to think Dad had thought about how he would have had to make a choice about how to lose Mom.

Instead he had time with her. It was challenging and difficult at times, but also filled with laughter. They had spent hours that last year sitting and holding hands. Although he never said it out loud, it was obvious Dad was very much aware their time together was limited. And I think deep within her, Mom knew also.

The next morning I went to get Dad to take him to the hospital to see Mom.

When I went in the back door, a towel bar that had been on the cabinet to the left of the back door was on the floor. The oven door was open. There was minor disarray in the dining room and living room.

Dad was in the TV room in his chair. He said he did not remember everything that happened, but he described a dream in which he was crawling through the dining room.

Best guess is he went to the kitchen for something and lost balance, grabbed at the towel rack, which broke, then tried to reach the oven – they were just a few feet apart.

He ended up on the floor either in the kitchen or made it to the dining room before falling and then crawled through the dining room and somehow managed to get back up. He did not have any scratches or pains, so I have no idea exactly what happened.

Dad and I made a visit to the hospital. The doctor came in while we were there and said Mom could go home.

That summer – the summer of 2009 – was rough.

Dad was beating the cancer and doing well until Mom and Dad got a notice form Adult Protective Services. There had been a concern filed about them – naming me as the perpetrator. Although my siblings had not seen our parents for about a year at that point, they were responsible for the allegation.

My parents' attorney called Adult Protective Services and explained my parents did not want the investigation to go forward.

State law says they had the right to make that decision. It also says once Adult Protective Services have been informed my parents did not want services, they were not to pursue any further action unless directed to do so by the Secretary of Social and Rehabilitation Services.

It was found unsubstantiated.

But the damage was done. Dad fell into a deep depression. He was worried this investigation would result in Mom being taken from him or they would both be forced to leave their home. They would not be able to stay at home without my help.

Dad never recovered from that depression. About two weeks after receiving the notification, he said he was tired of fighting them. He decided he would stay on the bed, stop eating, and die.

He did not completely stop eating, and I kept him going to appointments. I got him to eat and drink as much as I could. But that event – the threat of being forced out of their home was more than he could bear.

Within a couple of months he was talking about suicide. He wanted to just die. He kept saying he was tired of having to fight with my siblings.

We still had a lot of good times that summer, but Dad had given up.

On Friday, August 21, 2009, he told me he was dying. He said he could tell. He did not want to go to the hospital. He wanted to die at home.

The next day Mom and I were in Dad's room talking to him.

Mom said, "I love you."

Dad replied, "I love you, too."

"Are you okay?"

"No, I am not doing well."

"Keep good thoughts, and you will get better."

Through that weekend I fed Dad as much as he would eat. I kept him drinking as much as I could. And kept him warm.

Despite it being August in Kansas, a very hot month, he was cold. I kept a continuous supply of warm blankets. He had 13 blankets piled on him. Every 30 minutes to an hour, I would pull them back and put a warm blanket on him and cover him again. There was a space heater in his room going full blast.

I also kept his CD player going with his favorite music.

He did not want to watch television.

Monday, August 24, about 6 am, I found him non-responsive.

After Dad died, and I continued to care for Mom, I inherited not only the job of caregiving but also seeing the beauty in Mom.

It was part of why I never saw her as anyone other than the beautiful person she had always been.

I greeted her each day with, "Good morning, Beautiful."

It was not just to affirm her beauty, but it was keeping with the commandment to honor my parents....no exceptions.

I was checking Mom's pulse – part of my routine. I told her I was checking to see if she was still alive. She pinched me. I said, "Ow." She said, "We are alive."

January 2012

> Mom: Oh, God
> Me: I am Carol, not God.
> Mom: That is obvious.
> July 2010

> Mom got in a fret mode and just walked around talking – I did not always know who or what she was talking to.
>
> One day while in fret mode she said, "I just walk around talking to myself like I am out of my head."
>
> September 2010

> I helped Mom get her coat and gloves on to go run errands. Then she announced she had to go to the bathroom. I told her I wish she had thought of that before we go her ready.
>
> Her response, "I just got that way."
>
> December 2010

Carol Luttjohann

IMAGINARY FRIENDS

I went to change Mom's linens and clothes. She was facing the wall talking to what I used to refer to as one of her imaginary friends. When I started to take the blanket, she turned to me and protested. I told her I had to take it to wash it. She let go, then looked back at the wall and said, "I'm sorry. I was talking to someone else."

Imaginary friends showed up once in a while. As we were getting out of the car one day, Mom turned to her "friend" and asked if she should get out of the car. Her friend said she should. I told Mom I wished I could see her imaginary friends. She replied, "So do I. There's a lot of them, and they are really nice."

I often wondered if Mom's imaginary friends were her way of keeping people in her life. As happens all too often with people with dementia, people who had been a part of Mom's life did not see value in visiting her. They said she would not know them. Also, having imaginary friends helped her have some control over her life.

One person who asked about seeing Mom I encouraged until she asked, "Will she even know who I am?" When faced with that question, it was difficult for me to not feel the anger. I explained there was no predicting if Mom would know her name or not, but I did know Mom would love the visit. The person chose not to visit. She had the all too familiar attitude of "Why bother?"

The few that did visit Mom were always greeted with a big Mom smile. She loved to hold hands of visitors. And, of course, eat ice cream together.

I am not sure if I like calling Mom's imaginary friends hallucinations or not. I am sure there were times she was talking to someone specific – a friend or family member she missed having in her life.

A lot of times she talked with her friends on the telephone. I think her friends were a coping mechanism. They were never scary or uncomfortable for her. That is why I think they were familiar people visiting her or talking to her on a telephone.

One night I heard her in her bedroom talking. When I went to check, she was obviously on a phone call. She would talk, wait, talk. What was comical is she kept trying to get off the phone. She would say, "Well I have to go…" Pause. "I'm glad she was able to do that…" Pause. She did eventually end the call.

We got interrupted with a phone call one time while I was feeding her. She stopped, picked up the "phone," put it to her ear, and said, "Hello." Paused a moment. Then she said, "I'm eating right now, can I call you back?" Pause. "Okay, I will talk to you later." She went back to eating.

Although there was a time when I heard her having a conversation with herself:

Mom: What do you think?

Mom Response: About what?

Mom: Anything.

Mom Response: Nothing.

I asked who she was talking to. She replied, "Myself."

"Do you answer yourself?"

"Yes. That is how I know I get the right answer."

She never failed with quick comebacks when I asked about her talking to herself.

One time when I asked if she was talking to herself, she said, "Yes."

"What do you say to yourself?"

"Oh, Sweetie, you are so cute."

When helping her put on shoes and socks one day, I told her she had cute feet. She said that is because she talks to her feet.

I asked, "What do you say to your feet?"

<Looking at feet.> "How are you today? No sores. No corns. No pain. That's good." <Then turning to me.> "See, it works."

Mom's podiatrist attributed to the good shape her feet were in to managing diabetes, food massages to keep circulation good and plenty of lotion. But maybe it was really Mom talking to her feet that did the most good.

Her imaginary friends changed over time. And once in a while she got mad at one. It was in her last few months of life, she was talking to one of her friends and said, "Don't touch my… my….my… SOMETHING."

Whatever that something was, she definitely did not want it touched!

It was also evident her friends were familiar to her and knew me. I heard her tell a friend, "I'm doing just fine because my daughter is here. Carol takes good care of me."

As we moved closer to what were last final

days of life, her conversations with imaginary friends focused on memories of Dad and her parents. I believe she was talking to them and preparing for her journey to be with them.

But nothing replaces how her conversations with her friends affirmed many times she knew my name, loved me, and truly appreciated my caring for her so she could stay in her own home.

I think Mom's imaginary were a result of coping with how she was treated because of her illness. She needed them to keep in contact with people that she knew. Typically it sounded like she knew her imaginary friend.

There is a fine line of difference between attributing her friends to hallucinations and as a coping mechanism. But the question becomes would Mom have needed imaginary friends if, although dementia can be scary, her friends had not been more concerned about what Mom was able to do rather than what they expected from her?

Mom was not dementia. She was, is, and will always be my mom.

Mom, Clancy, and I were on the back porch. Mom got up and was walking around and kind of stumbled.

Me: What are you doing?

Mom: Almost falling.

Me: That is not good.

Mom: Almost is not as bad as being on the floor.

July 2010

We were on the back porch on a cool spring day. Mom was wrapped in a blanket and had a space heater pointed at her.

She said, "This is nice. It would be perfect if I had ice cream."

She got ice cream.

April 2010

> Mom was having a very good day. She did not like the bath aid.
>
> Mom to Aid: I don't like this nonsense. Stop that. 1….2….3…
>
> However she was happy with me cleaning her up and helping her changed clothes. She even helped some.
>
> August 2011

> Me: I need to help you get your seatbelt on.
>
> Mom: I might help, but I have to take it under advisement first.
>
> August 2010

> Mom: What are you doing?
>
> Me: Making a grocery store list for tomorrow.
>
> Mom: I want ice cream <pause> cookies <pause> and chocolate.
>
> Yes. She got them all.
>
> September 2010

Carol Luttjohann

TRIPS NEAR AND FAR AND EVERYTHING IN BEWTEEN

Mom enjoyed going places and doing things. She had all of her life, so we made trips – some in town events, some short, and a couple of longer ones. Just like Mom, Kathleen, John and I had done in summers many years ago.

A favorite was trips to Abilene, Kansas. That is where a Russell Stover factory is located. It's a little over an hour drive from our hometown of Topeka, Kansas. They also have a large candy store with lots of sugar free options, and they have ice cream. What more could Mom want?!

The first time we went it was pretty event free. She picked lots of candies for herself and some presents for friends at home. It was topped off with ice cream.

The second trip we stopped at a Cracker Barrel in Junction City along the way. They have wonderful vegetables that she loved. We also got a Kenny Rogers gospel CD. More music for Mom.

She was in her wheelchair on the second trip. When we got to the Russell Stover store, I wheeled her in. We were looking at the tables of candy. I turned back around and discovered she had walked in her chair over to her favorite section –the ice cream.

As usual, everyone in the store loved her. She was so sweet. She got her ice cream, and we went to check out. She told everyone she would be back in ten days. She finished her ice cream and started on some of the candy on the trip home. Giving her what she loved and loving watching her enjoy was always rewarding.

We also took a short trip periodically to Burlingame, Kansas – only about 30 minute drive. That is where the horses and burro lived.

Mom's former neighbor, Linda, does horse rescue. Mom and I would go visit the animals. She would pet them and watch them. She loved the interaction with the horses and burros. There were chickens and dogs also.

On one trip a horse kept trying to lick Mom. That was not tolerable to Mom. She moved. The horse would move. Finally she got far enough away and started petting another horse.

We made a couple of trips to Burns, Kansas and Newton, Kansas. Burns is a small town about 25 miles east of Newton. Newton is north of Wichita. Mom had cousins that lived in Burns, Kansas. Her cousin, Rosalie, and her husband, Frank, spent some time in a nursing home in Newton, Kansas.

One visit was for Rosalie's and Frank's anniversary. Mom and Rosalie (who also had dementia) sat at a table and talked as only they could do. They were sitting at a table eating cake. Rosalie turned to talk to her friend. When her back was turned, Mom ate Rosalie's cake.

Me: That is Rosalie's cake.

Mom: There's more over there <pointing at the refreshment table>.

We also made the trip for Thanksgiving in 2010. Rosalie's and Frank's daughter, Sandra, fixed the majority of the meal. We took a few things. We were joined by Sandra's son, Jim, and his son, Steven. It was a wonderful afternoon.

Mom was getting a bit fretful at one point, so I took her for a walk. It worked. Walking is good especially because of the diabetes. Exercise brings down blood sugar.

We made a couple of very short trips in town to the Historical Society. Mom used to volunteer with the Historical Society. She taught candle making in public schools. She was also involved with Ward-Meade a historical homestead in Topeka.

Mom and a group she was part of started Apple Fest that was held annually at Ward

Meade. It started as a focus on pioneer crafts. It grew. Once it had roots and was growing rapidly, the city decided to manage the project. Ward Meade is a city park.

At the Historical Society – the first time we went we toured the building. I took pictures of Mom looking at various things. We talked about what she could remember. Sometimes memories came back as she looked around.

I also took her to the Historical Society for Kansas Day in 2011 – the state's 150th year anniversary celebration. We went specifically for music. There was a bluegrass group. Mom was in her wheelchair, and we sat on the front row. She was engaged and loved the music.

The biggest trip we took was to San Antonio, Texas with a stop in Rockwall, Texas to see Sherry. Mom had been asking about Sherry. She wanted to see her. Sherry could not find time to come to Kansas, so we went to Texas Mom smiled when she saw Sherry.

She was not very talkative, but she enjoyed the visit.

We went to San Antonio, Texas to Morgan's Wonderland.

While other theme parks accommodate people with disabilities and/or special needs, Morgan's Wonderland was created with them in mind. This park was built to emphasize inclusion, so we want everyone to come and enjoy Morgan's Wonderland![1]

It is an awesome place! They limit the number of people at the park. Reservations are required. People with special needs do not always tolerate crowds.

Mom loved the merry-go-round. It has a ramp for access, then there were special "cars" that were accessible. They strapped Mom's Wheel chair in. And the car she was in also went in an up and down motion – just like the animals on poles. Because there are no lines, Mom was able to ride the merry-go-round four times without getting off.

We also rode the train. There are cars with ramps for wheelchair accessibility. Again, they strapped down the wheelchair so she could enjoy the ride. We walked around the lake. We played instruments in the outdoor musical area. We played on the playground equipment… because she could. We watched children play in the water area. It was wonderful.

There are cars – the kinds that run on a track, and riders can pretend they are driving. I wheeled Mom up a ramp to a landing. They swung the entire landing over behind a car, opened the back of the car and wheeled Mom onto it. She was strapped in, and we could ride the car along the track.

She also liked the sensory building. There were all kinds of things to see and do. There were nursing students volunteering that day. Gale was our guide in the building. Everyone that comes into the building has a volunteer that stays with them and helps them.

She also was able to get on the swings. Swings are accessible. She rolled up on a ramp and was locked down. Then a couple of volunteers moved the swing for her. And everywhere there were employees and volunteers who would use our camera and take pictures.

They thought of everything.

It was worth the long drive and three nights on the road.

But the last trip Mom made out was September 2012. Deanna and Chris and their dogs, Shattan and Mini, were camping at Lake Shawnee and invited Mom, Clancy, and me to come out to eat and visit.

Her arthritis kept her from being comfortable bending her knees, so getting her out was challenging.

I got help to get her in the car. We got her in her wheelchair –one that both arms could be removed. I took off both arms, and we turned her in her wheelchair and slid her across   the backseat. She sat with her legs out and a pillow at her head. She was semi-reclined and buckled in for the ride.

Chris and Deanna got her out and helped get her into a gravity chair. She sat by a campfire and looked out over the lake.

Mom <looking at fire>: Who did that?

Deanna: I did.

Mom: Good job.

She had yogurt with granola, pasta salad and chocolate and enjoyed being outside.

As it was getting dark, I took her home.

Deanna and Chris helped get Mom back in the car. Deanna came up with the idea to tip the wheelchair and slide Mom basically up the back of the chair as it tipped and into the car. It worked like a charm.

I gave her a bottle of Coke for her ingeniousness. Coke is her favorite.

When we got home, I called paramedics to

help get her back in the house safely. It is a free service they provide.

Mom loved her outing. It was great for her to be outside, sit by a fire, and look at the lake. She had a wonderful night's sleep. She was tired the next day also.

It was just two months later she died.

> Never give up.
> Make the effort.
> Make all the memories you can.
> You won't regret it.

[1]Morgan's Wonderland Website. – www.morganswonderland.com

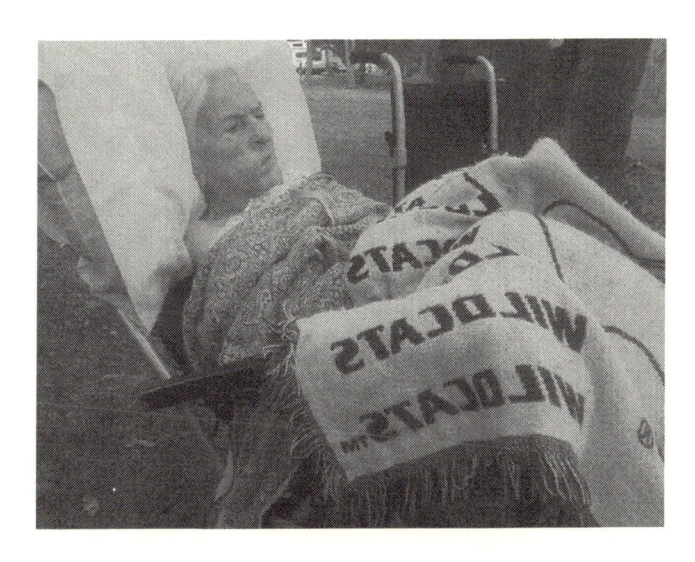

Mom's last outing: spending time at the lake with Chris, Deanna, Clancy, Shattan, Mini, and me. She had yogurt with granola – one of her favorites- pasta salad and chocolate. She is watching the campfire and looking out over the lake. Beautiful!
September 2012

The final chapter chronicles my last sixteen months with Mom.

There is some progression in her abilities and speech, but the strength she had throughout her life remained.

She was still a feisty lady who stood up for herself.

Most of all she never lost her love for ice cream.

Not everyone with dementia follows a path. Each follows their own.

Mom's communication and ability to understand remained strong. She knew what she wanted and asked for it.

My passion – keeping Mom at home- meant being able to always see the strengths that remained and loving her as she was.

Because she was, she is, and will always be my mother.

Carol Luttjohann

LUCKY DAUGHTER WONDERFUL MOMENTS

I will never understand my siblings, in-laws, and grandkids wanting to move Mom out of her home. It was if they gave up on her and decided they were not able to care for her at home, but that does not mean she should not stay at home. Dementia is scary, but that does not mean it is to be feared. There are stages of dementia, or at least that is what I have read, but Mom was supposedly in Stage 7 – the final stage in the fall of 2007, according to Kathy. That meant she was at the very end of the disease, but she lived more than five years after that.

A diagnosis of dementia does automatically make someone incompetent. Nor do signs of changes mean nothing can be done to help.

When Mom's diabetes and diet were under

control, she improved a lot. Throughout the years I cared for Mom, I was told countless times what a good job I did caring for her. Everyone fell in love with her and told me Mom was a sweet and wonderful lady with a great sense of humor.

During the four and one-half years I cared for her, I was truly blessed with not only her sense of humor and quick wit, but her sweet spirit. She told me frequently she loved me and how much she appreciated me taking care of her. She always knew me and knew my name. She was amazing.

It was July 6, 2011. I will never forget. She woke up and called me to her bed. By that time we were sharing the living room as our bedroom, so I was just a few feet from her. I went to her bed. She grabbed my hand. As she held it, she said, "I just want you to know how much I love you and appreciate you taking care of me. You are a wonderful person.

It's getting close to time for me to go."

This chapter is a journal of our last 16 months together in quips. Memories which are especially precious with the feisty lady that never lost her spirit and spunk.

****

July 6, 2011 I was helping Mom get out of the car.

Me: You need to help me.

Mom: You need to wait until I am ready.

****

Friday, July 22, 2011

Bath aid was giving Mom a massage

BA: Does that feel good?

Mom: Darn right that feels good.

****

Tuesday, July 26, 2011

Mom woke up hungry. Got her a "second supper", which she devoured. Then asked for ice cream. She was starting to get drowsy.

Me: Are you tired?

Mom: That's why I am closing my eyes.

****

Saturday, July 30, 2011

I was trying to help Mom eat. She was obviously tired.

Me: Are you hungry or do you want to rest a while first?

Mom: I'll tell you when I wake up.

****

Monday, August 1, 2011

I gave Mom a "Midnight" snack...two yogurts and a bowl of ice cream..

Me: Have you had enough ice cream?

Mom: (Laughing) You're funny.

She then opened her mouth for more - yep another bowl of ice cream. And then proclaimed she is cold. Spoiled, full, happy, and sleeping.

****

Thursday, August 4, 2011

I was helping Mom eat...

Me: Can you open your mouth?
Mom: Occasionally.
****

Monday, August 15, 2011
Me: Are you glad you are my mom?
Mom: I think so.
****

Thursday, August 25, 2011

I suggested that I make mashed potatoes and gravy, green beans, and broccoli for supper.

Mom replied, "How about I just eat ice cream and cake?"

She got her ice cream :)
****

Saturday, September 10, 2011

I was feeding Mom French Toast for breakfast and told her Braden and Luke from next door brought cookies over last night.

Mom: Can I have one now? Got a cookie for her and gave her a bite.

Mom: That is much better. How about some

ice cream, too? Mom had cookie and ice cream for breakfast - then ate more French Toast.

****

Monday, October 3, 2011

Me: I need to move you around so I can change the sheets and help you get cleaned up. You probably won't like it and will get mad.

(She usually did.)

Mom: Yes, but that's okay.

****

Saturday, October 15, 2011

Mom: I love you

Me: I love you, too.

Mom: Give me some ice cream.

****

Wednesday, October 26, 2011

Mom's long-time friend (over 70 years) called - I held phone to Mom's ear. Mom never said a word, but as soon as she heard Ruth's voice, she did her great big "Mom grin."

Definitely a connection.

****

Wednesday, December 7, 2011

Mom is not sleeping - first guess thirsty - nope, - second she is dry and clean - third hungry... tried oatmeal usually a staple, barely touched it... tried French toast a typical favorite.... nothing.

I gave her a chocolate chip cookie.

She said, "This is much better," with her beautiful Mom smile.

****

Monday, January 2, 2012

Fixed Mom a wonderful vegetarian dinner.

She had cole slaw, potato salad, mixed vegies, and fruit....she took a couple of bites, and said, "Do we have any ice cream?" Chocolate ice cream is always good. :)

****

Thursday, January 5, 2012

Beautiful sunshine day - moved Mom's bed right by the door so she can see outside and feel the sunshine. (Love the new storm door with full view.) And she is semi-sleeping and tapping her toes to John Denver music.

****

Tuesday, January 24, 2012

Me: Do you want a piece of chocolate?

Mom: Sure.

I unwrapped a Hershey's hug and started to put it in her mouth.

Mom: Did you wash your hands?

****

Sunday, January 29, 2012

Leaned over to check on Mom - she puckered up her lips, I leaned closer. She kissed me on the cheek and said, "I love you, Carol."

****

Sunday, February 5, 2012

Got Mom ready for lunch - starting feeding her tomato soup and grilled cheese. She smiled and said, "Thank you.

****

Monday, February 6, 2012

Gave Mom a foot massage followed by doses of chocolate.

Me: I sure do spoil you.

Mom: Keep it up.

****

Friday, February 10, 2012

Hospice Chaplain was here.....Mom slept most of the time. When she woke up, she held his hand and ate ice cream (surprise surprise). Then asked about praying, and she became very alert and thanked him several times. Some things are still very important to her...it's fascinating what she hears, understands, and how she responds.

****

Wednesday, February 22, 2012

Physical therapist came today - Mom sat on the edge of her bed for almost 30 minutes. That is a goal - get her sitting on bed and hopefully then in wheelchair. Doing all we can to keep her comfortable, happy, and strong.

****

Thursday, February 23, 2012

Hospice Social Worker came today....told me they all wished all   the families they work with were as good at care as I am. :)

****

Sunday, February 26, 2012

Used the last of the chocolate chip cookie dough and made two cookies. Gave Mom a bite of one (fully intending we would each eat one). She opened her mouth for more... Greater love hath no daughter than to feed her mother both warm chocolate chip cookies and instead eat a banana herself.

****

Tuesday, February 28, 2012

Mom: Do we have any cookies? Gave her one of her cookies.

Mom: This is cold.

She just finished three fresh baked chocolate

chip cookies.

****

Tuesday, March 13, 2012 Mom is up in her wheelchair, spent an hour on the porch, ate ice cream, gave Clancy treats.

While feeding her ice cream, she looked at me and said, "You sure are a cute baby." She also responded to neighbor calling her by name - not a frequent event, but does happen. She is exhausted, but inside and still in the chair for now.

****

Thursday, March 15, 2012

Me: Do you want some apple pie and ice cream?

Mom: That would make my day!

****

Friday, March 16, 2012

Another milestone: Took Mom for a walk today - instead of just sitting on porch. She tried to "walk" in the wheelchair. Inconsistent and difficult, but she was trying. Walked two blocks. She is exhausted!

Although communication is not as good today as it was the last couple of days.

She is happy!

****

Thursday, March 22, 2012

I was feeding Mom Mint Oreo Cookie ice cream.

Me: Do you like eating ice cream?

Mom: Yep.

Me: You get everything you want.

Mom: That's right.

****

Friday, March 30, 2012 Another milestone - got Mom out today - in the car. She was able to go in the Party America store with me to get a balloon for her birthday. :) Then to lunch. That was all she could handle. She was tired. Home for a short rest, then she wanted to go outside, so she sat on the porch while I got the yard ready for party tomorrow. Ended with giving her some ice cream and her looking me in the eye and saying, "I love you, Carol." Now she is snoring. :)

****

Monday, April 2, 2012

Getting Mom cleaned up which can be challenging.

Mom: You stop that.

Me: I need to get you clean. Gave her a short break and went to finish.

Mom: I said stop that. If you don't do what I say, we are going to have real problems.

So glad she is staying happy and spunky. I love my energetic, stand up for herself, not put up with nonsense Mom.

****

Friday, April 13, 2012

Me: How are you doing today?

Mom: I'm feeling a lot better. What are we

doing today?

Me: Going to the grocery store.

Mom: Okay.

****

Saturday, May 12, 2012

Took Mom out to eat breakfast for Mother's Day.

Got her out of car and into wheelchair, then have to pull her up to a sitting (instead of slouching) position.

Me: I need to pull you up so you will sit straight.

Mom: No

Me: Yes (as I pulled her up)

Mom: (shaking finger at me) Now you listen to what I say.

Had a great time with breakfast and she ate well. Now home and sleeping.

****

Tuesday, May 15, 2012

Been outside for almost 5 hours now. Asked

Mom if she is getting tired. She replied, "No, but I am hungry for ice cream."

****

Thursday, June 14, 2012

This morning I made Mom her morning oatmeal with blueberries and cinnamon today.

However, while I was letting it set to a cool a bit, she told her "friends," "I am getting ready to eat some ice cream." She had ice cream for breakfast.

****

Sunday, July 1, 2012

My beautiful mom woke up and I asked if she wanted to go outside to eat breakfast. She said, "Yes." I went to get things to clean her up and get her outside. When I got back to her bed, she grabbed my hand, held it very tightly, and said, "I love you." She kept hold of my hand and went back to sleep. We will go outside later. :)

****

Friday, July 27, 2012

Mom: I'm cold.

Me: I'll get you a blanket. I get the blanket and cover her with it.

Mom: It's not warm.

I put another blanket in the dryer, take it out a few minutes later, take off the "wrong" blanket, and cover her with the warm blanket.

Mom: That's better.

****

Tuesday, July 31, 2012

Mom spent almost 6 hours in her wheelchair walking backwards most of the time. Then I would put her back in place to walk some more. Eating a LOT of food. Drinking water, juice and oost. She talks about Carol a lot to her "friends."

But most of all- very, very happy. She is exhausted.

****

Sunday, August 5, 2012

Gave Mom a warm blanket...

Me: Does that feel good?

Mom: Yep

Me: Do you like warm blankets?

Mom: Yep <<<eyes closing, very drowsy>>>

Me: Are you tired?

Mom: zzzzzzzzzzzzzzzzzzz

The wonderful sounds of Snoring

****

Monday, August 6, 2012

Mom: Are we going outside?

Me: We can if you want. You are in charge.

Mom: That's good.

****

Friday, August 24, 2012

Deanna came and stayed with Mom and Clancy for a while this morning.

Deanna: You raised a wonderful daughter. Carol is a good person. She loves you and takes good care of you.

Mom: I know

Then she fell asleep. She is amazing.

****

Sunday, September 2, 2012

Got Mom in her wheelchair and into bathroom for a "shower."

Put several layers of blankets (hospital white) and towels to absorb the water -usually enough. However, today she said how good the warm water felt and was rubbing herself to work the lather up with the soap herself. HUGE mess, but worth it. She felt clean and was trying to do it herself. Worth all the mess and all the extra laundry!

****

Friday, September 28, 2012

Took Mom to Lake Shawnee Campgrounds to spend the afternoon with friends who are camping. She sat in a gravity chair they have, ate lots of pasta salad, yogurt, and chocolate, was very conversational, and smiled a lot.

Wonderful outing!

****

Tuesday, November 6, 2012

Mom has been sleeping a lot - UTI kicking her butt - antibiotics are starting to work.

She woke up.

Told her I have quiche, applesauce, and no bake cookies for her.

She ate some applesauce, ate some quiche, closed her mouth. Asked if she wanted more quiche.

She replied, "Chocolate."

She is eating cookies.

****

Saturday, November 17, 2012

Mom's eyes are closed - could not tell if sleeping or not.

Me: Are you awake?

Mom (with eyes closed and very quietly): No

****

Thursday, November, 29, 2012

My beautiful mother is reunited with Dad.

In the last moments of life, she squeezed my hand. She smiled, and she told me she loves me.

She knew I was there, and that means more than anything.

AFTERWORDS

I am passionate about caring for people in their own homes. I believe strongly that elderly have the right to make choices about their own lives, including where and how they live.

There is a need for better supportive services to keep people at home. The cost is much lower to keep people at home than to place them in out of home facilities. Dementia care units run between $7,000 and $10,000 a month. Keeping Mom at home was under $2,000 a month. Costs for the four and one-half years at home was closer to $108,000 total less than two years in out of home placement.

Respite services required Mom to go to a facility. I did that once. I spent a lot of time with her at the facility. I got a lot done, but more beneficial to me and to Mom would have been a couple of all days with her at home. At least that should be an option.

A gripe I have about Home Health and Hospice sounds trivial on the surface. It is about being on time and following through. That was challenging for most. Aids were scheduled for 3 pm but would show up anywhere from noon to 5 pm. Nurses would say morning and come at 6 pm.

I know – the caregiver is at home, so it is okay to not keep a schedule. They will there anyway, right?

That is true they are at home, but that does not mean the caregiver does not keep a schedule with someone they are caring for.

It does not mean the caregiver did not plan on the aid being there at 2:00 p.m. so she could run an errand.

I had it happen many times.

I told a friend I would be by her office at 2:15 p.m. because the aid was to be here at 2:00

p.m. When the aid was late, it snowballed. I was late so my friend was late...

But there is also a very significant reason to stay on schedule. Practically everything in a caregiver's life is outside their control – progression of disease, good or bad day for the patient, and so much more. When aids / nurses / other health care professionals randomly change schedules or do not show up at all, it creates a great deal of stress. The hospice / home health professionals have become one more "thing" that the caregiver cannot depend on, one more "thing" outside of their control instead of someone they can depend on.

The last two aids we had were wonderful.

The two came together to care for Mom because it was difficult to move her with her arthritis. They were kind and gentle with her. They considered her comfort most important. They got it.

And, of course, our most favorite nurse,

Deanna. A master of caring for people and their families. She included pets in caring for families because they are family.

And, most of all, we need to change how we care for people with dementia. It is changing, but slowly.

Dementia is scary, but I think a big part of that mindset comes from all the focus on what might happen with someone with dementia.

It has to sound devastating to raise money for research for prevention and hopefully cures or treatments.

I am not even going to pretend I think dementia is a good thing, but I wonder how many people get less than adequate treatment and / or care because families see no hope and just let the disease take its course.

I cannot even tell you how many times people told me they did not visit Mom because she would not know them anyway. They did not think she would remember they were there.

They rationalized it was okay to not visit her because it would not make a difference to her. Bluntly, that is bull shit.

Mom was always glad to have visitors. Although she was not always able to remember names, she knew people. It made a difference to Mom. Because information focuses on all of what might happen, there is fear of being around people with dementia.

Dementia robs people of their memory. They lose abilities to smile and talk. They lose ability to walk. We have heard all the horror of it. But the problem is the information scares people, and it is not applicable to every person with dementia.

Mom never stopped smiling. She remained verbal - not as active and coherent all the time, but she was able to talk and ask for ice cream until the day she died.

She was not able to walk, but, for her, it was because of arthritis.

When she had difficulty using silverware, I gave her a lot of finger foods and helped feed her when she needed help. There were times she started eating with a spoon, and then finished her oatmeal using her fingers. So what!

Get past expectations and rules and allow people to do the most they can. And when she was no longer able to feed herself at all, I helped her.

But here is another question....why should it have mattered if Mom knew anyone's name?

My blunt reaction is how selfish...if she cannot remember "your" name. She still deserved to be treated with dignity and respect. Remembering is an expectation that people with dementia have a great deal of difficulty meeting.

Why should that matter?

What if the expectations change to there are no expectations? Do not expect people with dementia to remember names or have all the skills they used to have. But, also, don't expect people with dementia to be combative and totally helpless. Instead allow them to be who they are – who they have always been. Granted I was there every day all day and night, but Mom never forgot my name. She always knew me.

Dementia might be scary, but do not be afraid of people who have dementia.

Claudia Jean McInstosh Luttjohann was not an old lady with dementia...she was, she is, and she will always be my mother.

Mom's care was in the shop for repair. We were driving my truck. She was short and barely reached the seat. She backed up to it and said, "Throw my feet in."
March 2011

A bath aid was doing Mom's nails and said, "Your nails are going to look so pretty."
Mom replied, "I am pretty."
August 2011

I asked Mom if she wanted to go visit Kathleen.
Mom: <Blank stare>
Me: Are you going to talk or just stare at me?
Mom: I think I will just stare at you.
December 2010

ABOUT THE AUTHOR

Carol Luttjohann cared for her parents, Leo and Claudia, from May 2008 to August 24, 2009 when Leo died.

She then continued to care for Claudia until she died November 29, 2012. Carol lived in her parents' home with them so they could remain where they wanted to be.

She earned her Bachelor of Arts at Ottawa University in Ottawa, KS, a Master of Religious Education at Southwestern Baptist Theological Seminary in Fort Worth, Texas, and her Master of Social Work at Washington University in St Louis.

She lives in Topeka, Kansas with her dog, Clancy Jasper and cat, Delilah Lucille.

She can be reached through email at claudiasplace@gmx.com, and you can find more pictures and "Mom-isms" on her blog at http://carolluttjohann.wordpress.com/

Made in the USA
Charleston, SC
28 September 2013